A PARAMEDIC'S DAZE

FROM THE HUMBLE BEGINNINGS OF A PARAMEDIC'S 40 YEAR JOURNEY

DAVID BRADBURY

Copyright © 2025 by David Bradbury
All rights reserved.
ISBN: 978-1-7644288-0-4
No part of this publication may be reproduced, distributed, or transmitted in any form or by any means, including photocopying, recording, or other electronic or mechanical methods, without the prior written permission of the publisher, except as permitted by U.S. copyright law. For permission requests, contact Dave via email, braddersemail@yahoo.co.uk
For privacy reasons, some names, locations, and dates may have been changed.
Book cover by Getcovers.com
1st edition 2025

DEDICATION

This book is dedicated to all the people who tirelessly work for the good of others in often difficult and inhuman conditions. They miss sleep, meals, weekends, kid's growing up, Christmas's and life, in the delivery of care to others. On this basis the dedication also extends to my daughter Emily, following in her dad's footsteps, my daughter Chloe, and my son Michael. Sorry isn't enough for all the time spent away from your childhoods. I just hope and prey those who received my attention appreciated just what I gave up.

To Donna, for reasons which will become clear. And of course, to Mary Stowe, God bless her soul, without whom my adventures and this book would never have begun.

Dave Bradbury has worked in pre-hospital care for nearly 40 years, to create a lifetimes worth of experiences that have been immortalised to the pages of this book. Paramedic's tales are certainly not a new thing, but every author has a different take and perspective on what they have seen and captured, and how they relate it to the reader. 'A Paramedic's Daze' is the first snapshot in a series of ongoing writings of Dave's experiences seen from the eyes of a young, green ambulanceman through to experienced paramedic on the streets of Birmingham, from the eighties through to the naughties.

Ambulances, cars, motorbikes and helicopters feature within tales of laughter, woe, death and down right destruction. So come and laugh, cry, sigh and howl with him as he takes you through his journey....

FOREWORD

Have you ever realised that whatever you do for a job, whoever you're partnered with, and whatever opportunities have come your way, good or otherwise, these things happened because you were introduced some time before to someone, who knew someone, who introduced you to someone, who gave you the idea, who ultimately led you in some way to your job, your wife, your husband, your best mate, your car, your house? The Chaos Theory; and so the Butterfly Effect is derived; the theoretical example of a hurricane's formation being initiated from a distant butterfly who flapped its wings several weeks before, and whose movements accentuated over time. Everything we are or do is as a result of being in the right place, at the right time, or perhaps in the case of the unfortunates, the wrong place at the wrong time. Left to our own devices, and without contact with others, the internet, media or communication, we'd only advance as far as our instincts would allow. Well, that's my perspective on me. The following tales of laughter, sadness, irony and excitement are all true, as they actually happened……although many names have been altered.

CHAPTER 1.
THE HUMBLE BEGINNINGS.

I never set out to join the ambulance service. Like so many of my colleagues who have 20 years or more under their belts, I drifted in; the product of being in the right place at the right time; knowing the right people, and being given the idea, which, following a period of rejection, grew in my mind as the acorn does into the oak tree.

I'd been working for a large insurance company, collecting premiums door to door in some of the inner city and poorer parts of Birmingham in the mid 1980's. As a fresh, inexperienced 18 year old, the offer of doubling my wages from the factory I'd been in had given me no contest. Cleaner work, wearing a suit and working my own hours was infinitely more attractive than getting up at 5am six days a week, and spending most of my time covered in oil and grease, and being bullied by the works foreman, a young Indian guy, only a few years my senior, but with a power crazy ego and little else to his credit.

In the days before direct debit, and internet payments, paying life and endowment insurance premiums weekly to the man from 'The Pru', or 'The Vic', as I was known, was common place, especially amongst lower socio-economic classes of the areas I used to work. These were people whose pay came as cash in a packet once a week from their employers. Even the ambulance service paid the ambulance men and women the same way. My inexperience of life meant I had no concept of the risk I put myself in daily, walking around these areas of high unemployment and where crime was common place, dressed in a suit and carrying a black book. I might just as well have had a sign above my head stating 'Rob Me, I'm carrying loads of cash'!

But typical of my impulsive, unsettled character, a couple of years down the line, boredom struck. The good wages, clean conditions and working the hours I wanted weren't enough. I needed something else but hadn't got a clue what. I don't even remember at that time putting effort into hunting a new job and career. I just knew I needed something. I'd always been jealous of my eldest brother Stuart, who, from a young age, knew where his destiny lay in interior design. I recall him lecturing to me when I was about 14 years old that I had to hurry up and decide what I wanted to do before it was too late. Too late for what? I didn't know, but I feared it all the same. And at that age, in school, I dropped some subjects and took others, still with no idea whether these were good areas that would help me or not. Today of course, it doesn't matter if young people don't know what career direction they want to proceed in. They can happily move from job to job until they find their niche. Indeed many employers now realise the advantages of employing mature people in their 30's, 40's and 50's tempting these individuals to change jobs and start new careers. They bring a wealth of maturity, worldly experience, settled character and presence.

One of my regular collections was from Mary. Mary was married to John, as she called him, or 'Jack' as I later knew him. I didn't know it at the time, but these two people provided a pivotal turning point in my life from which all the rest of my subsequent adventures stem, and to which I owe an immeasurable debt of gratitude.

Mary was a woman in her late fifties when I first met her. A housewife, she was short in height with jet black, shoulder length curly hair and a round face that always had a smile on it. She'd often be wearing a pink 'pinny'; a sort of skirt cover that tied at the back and let me know that she'd been busy with the cleaning or the cooking, by the presence of a dusting of flour, or a tin of furniture polish peeking out of the front pocket. Occasionally, plastic hair curlers adorned the top of her head, covered over with a pink head scarf, and providing her with a degree of embarrassment and apology that she should dare to look this way to me. Of course, to me it didn't matter. It made Mary who she was.

Mary saw no bad in anybody or anything, and was always cheery and bright, even on the dullest of days. I used to think that she didn't have a grasp on reality sometimes; that she wasn't aware of the bad things I was seeing in the papers, like the murders, the robberies and rising unemployment. She reminded me of the character, Florence Johnson, played by Hilda Braid, as the dotty mother of Wolfie's girlfriend, Shirley in the 1970's UK sitcom 'Citizen Smith'. But she was a steadfast loyal wife to Jack, and a through and through Brummie girl, always having his tea on the table at the right time, buying his favourite brand of cigars, and making sure his house was always clean and tidy with the pantry stocked and the gardens neat.

Mary and Jack lived in a two storey block of council maisonettes in Nechells, Birmingham. They were in the shadow of 3 much larger tower blocks, and the area was very much 'inner city'. They'd moved in when the blocks were first built, during the 1960's, getting preferential placement due to Jack working for what was then The Birmingham Fire and Ambulance Service. When new, the area bustled with fresh faces enjoying the freedom of the more open spaces and the new social housing provided for them to rent from Birmingham Council. The alternative had been the slums of the 'back to back' terraces of Aston and Handsworth, other local suburbs, where four houses would share a single outside toilet, known as the 'lavvy'. The women all did their washing on the same day, lighting a fire under the wash tub, using washboards and wringing out with a mangle. The old fire grates would need 'blacking' weekly and it would not have been uncommon for a family of 9 or 10 children to be living in these often 2 bedroomed houses.

In these new 60's housing projects, inner city Birmingham land was at a premium, so building went in an upwards direction and tower blocks and flats sprung up in abundance. In the early days, crime was relatively unheard of and a real community spirit developed where the men went out to work and the women took their turns in cleaning the communal hallways, and each looked out for the welfare of the others. Children played in safety on the streets, and this was a nice place to live. But twenty years on, this same place had become the slum it replaced. The main of the dwellings held good honest people; people who'd been there from the start. And the remainder? Others with significantly lower moral and ethical standards. Drugs, prostitution, crime, and an element of uncaring was taking over. The once open grassed areas were now littered with used drug paraphernalia and were avoided as places where street robberies took place, usually to fund the drug issues. Loud music and barking dogs emulated from the tower block balconies. Used nappies, spilling bin bags and the sickly aroma of Jeyes Fluid now filled the hallways where once there had been routine, pride and polish.

Despite all this, Mary's was one regular call I used to look forward to, saving it until late afternoon when my round was nearly finished and I could relax with the sandwich and the cup of tea made with sterilised milk that Mary used to have waiting for me. We used to chat about all sorts, but the conversation often relegated towards her neighbours, what business they'd been up to, and other such gossip. Looking back, Mary used to look forward to my visits as much as I did, giving her the opportunity to tell me all the nitty gritty she'd obtained since my last visit.

"I see Mrs Cotton at 47s kicked 'er 'usband out agen. That'll be the third time this month" She'd say, continuing with, "Mind you, I'm not surprised. Always drunk 'e is. It's a bleedin' shame fer them babbies ya know," or "the Police was round next door this mornin' agen. A right bloody noise there was. Shoutin' and screamin'. They ended up taking 'im away with 'andcuffs on".

"Who did they arrest?" I'd asked,

"Bobby. Ya know Bobby. Always in trouble with the law" She gazed upwards, turning her head to the side slightly, as if day dreaming. "I remember 'im as a babby. Lovely curly blonde 'air 'e 'ad".

"Ah him. Yes I know" I agreed. But I didn't have a clue who she was on about. It was just easier to agree. She continued;

"He wuz all trussed up like a chicken 'e was. I don't think 'e was very 'appy neither. Ya should 'ave 'eard 'is bleedin' language! Shockin' it was."

This was the stage in my career that I often started to develop the ability to respond to this sort of conversation in all the right places, at all the right times, with all the right words of 'O really?', 'ah, I see' and 'hmm, that's terrible', or some such response, without actually consciously listening to Mary, because I wasn't really interested, but was far too polite to say anything else. This skill was to prove invaluable for my, as yet, unknown future career.

I knew Jack to be of a similar age to Mary, but for over 2 years, collecting their insurance premiums fortnightly, I rarely met him, forming most of my opinion of him from what Mary would say, which was very little. He was an ambulanceman, working at the local Henrietta Street depot in Hockley, Birmingham, and was usually on 'late' shifts when I called round for his insurance from Mary. When I finally met him, and had chance to chat with him, the reason seemed clear why Mary didn't tell me much about him. They had a very traditional marriage where chauvinism seemed to play a big part. He went to work to earn the crust; she stayed at home and kept the house. He didn't ask her about how the floor cleaning had gone that day or what the price of potatoes was, and neither did he ever tell her about his work experiences either. 'Never the twain shall meet', and they didn't. But some of Jack's almost secretive days at the ambulance station were to shield Mary from the horrors of the death and destruction that her husband had been dealing with. They were from a bygone era, where post traumatic stress disorder didn't seemingly exist, and ambulancemen of the day were mainly ex military men who were all told to toughen up following harrowing jobs.

On 21st November 1974 Jack attended the Birmingham pub bombings. 21 people lost their lives to horrendous blast injuries. 182 were injured. The scene was one of total devastation with many victims killed instantly. Jack's experiences of that one night alone changed him. He never discussed any of it with Mary. Not one thing.

Early in 1987, I called round to collect from Mary as usual. She astutely noticed that I wasn't my usual bubbly self and in her words, 'looked right pissed off'.

"Whats the marra, bab?" she asked, placing a thick, ham salad sandwich and a left over Christmas mince pie in front of me. She turned back to the singing kettle, pouring into a battered tea pot looking like it was old when it had been used at The Somme. Out came the sterilised milk, and my now half eaten sandwich was joined by a mug of traditional Birmingham sweet milky tea. My girlfriend's mother, Vi, had introduced me to this 'delicacy' some two years before, and it had virtually taken me all this time to be able to tolerate it.

"I don't know Mary," I replied with a glum tone. "I'm fed up with this job. I'm bored, but what worries me is I haven't got the faintest idea what I want to do."

By now, Mary had joined me at the table, as she often did. But in all the time I knew her, she would pour hospitality in my direction but would never partake in my presence herself. I later saw the same with Jack. His meals were always prepared and served immaculately and she would often stand and watch him eat in silence but would always eat on her own, in the kitchen, and never in front of her husband, except on Sunday, where the traditional roast was always served, often with the family coming round. But this never appeared to me to be 'behaviour'. It was devotion. They loved each other dearly. She wasn't down trodden, or put down. Jack only ever spoke of her with affection. She was his queen to look after and provide for, and he her king to worship.

"Why don't you become an ambulanceman?" she spoke, breaking a short period of silence while I was eating. For once I heard her. Mary's comment summed up her innocence, her naivety, her almost stupidity. I pondered between final mouthfuls my reply. I wanted to say how bloody stupid a suggestion that was; and how, if she couldn't come up with anything better then not to bother. Here was me, a spotty teenager, inexperienced in life, who hated the site of blood and couldn't cope with panic and mayhem, having the suggestion of becoming an ambulanceman, and doing all these very things I knew I couldn't do. But Mary's demeanour, and my compassion fitted perfectly.

"Oh I couldn't do that," I replied, wrinkling up my face in a sort of suggestion of horror.

"Why not?" she said, with a complete look of such sweet innocence. "John's been doing it for over 20 years". Her suggestion was obviously that if her husband, a veteran who completed his national service in the British army, went on to work on the railways before now entering his third decade having dealt with Birminghams worst death and destruction then clearly, this 20 year old, wet-behind-the-ear oik with a couple of O'levels, one in biology mind you, could obviously do the same. Her idea was preposterous. It was ridiculous. There was no way on God's earth that I could ever, or would ever deal with death, mutilation and all that blood guts and gore. So having finished my feed I thanked Mary heartily and left to complete my round for the day.

But Mary had started something. In all her perceived innocence she had laid a seed; a seed that was to become the adventure for the next 40 years of my life. I started to think that maybe the idea of dealing with all these things I thought I feared wasn't such a bad one after all. Over the next few days, I day dreamed about what it might be like; the excitement, the adventure, the adrenaline. But pah, it was probably just a pipe dream.

My next visit to Mary's was a morning call that I'd arranged with her as I'd taken on someone else's insurance round for a few weeks and needed some slight rearrangement. We again sat down with the cursory sandwich and cuppa, but this time the conversation was very different. I'd been thinking about what she'd suggested, I told her, and wondered if I could pop back later for a chat with her husband. I'd sort of expected her to be condescending and wondered why the change of heart. But not Mary. She was so matter-of-fact about my question, it was almost like she knew I'd ask it, like it was the most natural thing in the world.

"Well, John's had a meeting with the gaffer today so he'll be back about five, if you wanna pop back."

"Great," I replied with enthusiasm, "I'll be back later then."
I'd met Jack only a couple of times before, and they were quick fleeting glances. When he was home, his place was in the lounge, where he would sit in front of the tv, or be model making on the dining table, Mary only joining him in the evenings. His time in the kitchen was to eat, before resuming to the back lounge. It was just the way they liked it. To me, this room was almost sacred. Because I only ever saw Mary, I'd never been in there and wondered what it was like. In the same way that as a child I dreamed about what it was like to stand on the shop keepers side of the counter, and how different the perspective on things would be. And on those couple of brief momentary encounters with Jack, I'd hardly been able to form an opinion of him. I was part of Mary's world; in the same group as the rent man, and the gas meter man, so Jack had only ever given me a polite nod, or a quiet 'allo mate,' as he briefly popped into the kitchen for something while I was there.

But my eyes were to be opened wide to Jack, as I did indeed call back later that afternoon. A little nervous, and apprehensive of what to expect, I was soon put at ease. Mary greeted me and I was led to the lounge; mans territory! Jack stood up and reached out a hand for me to shake. He was of a similar height to me, ultra clean shaven with silvering wavy hair, and a vague smell of Old Spice aftershave. He'd clearly recently stepped out of the bath and was now dressed in a check shirt and brown tie done up, and complemented with brown trousers, neat slippers and a cream heavy cardigan with big brown leather buttons. I sensed none of this was for me, but his militaristic background meant he always dressed this way when relaxing at home. Like my grandad, I guessed he'd still wear a shirt and tie to clean the car or mow the lawns. His face had a welcoming but stern feel to it, almost like he had once been a hard man, a tough leader who took no prisoners, but in his maturity had mellowed, maybe through the addition of his grandchildren who I knew to be very young through Mary.

"Have a seat", Jack said in a gruff voice, looking me in the face. "Mary tells me you want to join The Ambulance Service". He leaned over to the table beside him, took out a cigar from the packet and proceeded to light it. He relaxed back into the chair and settled for my answer.

"Well, yes sir I'm thinking about it". I didn't know what to refer to him as; Jack? John? Sir? And being too afraid to ask, I didn't, avoiding having to refer to him by name at all, and deciding on the initial respectful route of sir. Jack was a Leading Ambulanceman or LA as they were known at that point. He was a shift leader, which in my eyes made him almost as high as the Chief Ambulance Officer. I would go on to get to know Jack very well. He commanded more respect from the blokes at Henrietta Street Station, than probably anyone I've met before or since, his secret being fair, reasonable and always fighting for his men and their welfare. He didn't care too much for the new breed of management. Oh, he respected their rank, but not many of them as people, and didn't care too much either of their new style of running 'his' station. Jack was old school alright, but from the same school where common sense, logic, reasoning and humanism come from. If one of his blokes needed time off for his mother's hospital appointment, Jack would give it, and cover the consequences. If another man screwed up, Jack would ball him out and that would be the end of it. And people respected him for it. If they were off sick, then they were genuinely sick, not pulling the wool, and if Jack couldn't give them the leave they wanted, they knew he'd busted his gut trying, and accepted it with no moans or complaints.

Jack and I chatted for hours. Every question I asked, we discussed until we'd exhausted it, and every question led to another two popping up. True to her hospitality, Mary kept the cups of tea and sandwiches coming thick and fast. My bladder took a severe beating that evening as it filled and filled but there was no time to use the toilet; too many questions were looming, and besides, asking to use the bathroom seemed impolite, until that point where it would burst. Finally, I left their place at gone two in the morning, having chatted openly about what the job entailed, its ups and downs, high points and lows. Jack clearly lived and breathed the service, and proudly so. But this modest man not once flew his own flag; not once did he recount any jobs he did, and not once did he tell me what a hero he'd been, saving countless lives. These would subsequently die with him, when he passed on many years later. I often wonder as I write this, what fantastic stories he would have been able to tell, had he been inclined.

By the time I left, I was hooked. What Mary had started, Jack had completed with such an enthusiastic and natural way. That was it, I was going to join the Ambulance service and become an ambulance man.

My first attempt at trying to join the ambulance service was met with a negative response. I'd sent an application in the day after Jack and I had had our mammoth chat. And a week later, I was notified that West Midlands Ambulance Service wouldn't consider my application until I was 21. This was three months away. I could have just bided my time but impulse took me to leave and try a few other jobs while I waited. Of course, in my one track mind, I was going to get in, period. To fail was not something I'd optioned. So, in the space of the next nine months (for the application process took this long), I sold pensions, mortgages and hospitality, worked a bar in a hotel and provided static security. Then in October 1987, following the selection process, I finally received my start date for the ambulance service. I was to report to The Station Officer of Henrietta Street depot at 0900 sharp on the 5th, to collect my uniform and a vehicle and travel to Wolverhampton for training. Could I possibly have had any idea what lay ahead? Adventures, laughter, tears, sadness, frustration and opportunity. No, I didn't give it a thought, and neither did I care. At 21, I was interested in the moment, not the future.

Henrietta Street Ambulance Station, Hospital Street, Birmingham, was to form a foundation of four decades of experience, providing in some shape or form, prehospital care to the sick, injured, lame and plain mad. That's many years of *experiences*. Dressed in smog coated bricks, this big, dark, drab, encroaching building was so typical of the style of medical buildings built in the same era. Sited just on the outskirts of Birmingham city centre, it housed memories, characters, noises and ghosts. Jack used to say that when he was alone in the station on nights, in the days when traffic ceased beyond midnight and all that remained was the deafening silence; silence enough to hear the proverbial pin drop, he could hear footsteps along the corridor. And when he'd been down to the bottom of the garage, known as 'the graveyard', he returned to the station to find something had moved, or a light was turned on in a room where he knew it hadn't been on earlier. And there was only him in the building……

Ghosts were hardly surprising though. The fleet of ambulances both current and past, had seen the last breath taken by thousands of poor individuals ranging from birth to centenarians and beyond. Heart attack, cancer, disease, shot, stabbed, burnt, run over, crushed, decapitated and mutilated. They'd seen it all. There was no form of death they hadn't. Blood, vomit, shit, and every other bodily fluid had been liberally smeared on their floors, walls and ceilings, and there were times when they resembled the canvas of the 5 year old child's spatter painting. Then opposite to the station on one side of Summer Lane was the old hospital, built and demolished several hundred years ago. How many had died of the consumption there? And the exit from the station saw the ambulances drive past the old mortuary to the hospital, a building which has remained empty and spooky since way before my time. Like I say, a few unaccountable noises and occurrences in the dead of night were not really a surprise.

I kept in regular contact with Jack and Mary for years, from that fateful moment back in 1987 when Mary's off the cuff suggestion changed my life forever. I went round to see them both at home every few months, and always at Christmas where we exchanged gifts. Of course, before he retired, I also regularly saw Jack at work when both of us happened to be on shift. In the early 90's, Jack took retirement at the age of 65. I wondered how he would cope and what he would do. This veteran hero had lived and breathed the ambulance service for decades, but unlike many of the guys, he wasn't a golfer and had little in the way of hobbies. When we spoke about his plans for retirement casually one day, he just said that him and Mary were looking forward to spending more time with the family, and when I asked, they didn't have any plans to travel as so many people do when they get their pension. A month's cruise in the Med, a world tour, or family trip to Florida and Disneyland were not in their remit. Mary and Jack were home birds; they lived in Nechells and loved it. And post retirement, Mary would still be found down at the local shops most mornings buying her bread and sterilised milk, the laundrette once a week, bingo on a Tuesday lunchtime and Alum Rock High Street for the weekly shop on a Saturday morning. The only difference now being that Jack would be in tow. I almost felt sorry for him, and his retirement was definitely the end of an era. Things wouldn't be the same any more.

For the first few months, Jack would call into the station about once a week when he was in town shopping. He'd bought himself a new, but second hand, car, and he appeared happy. He had good health, rosy cheeks and a skip in his step, but I got the impression from him, that his visits to the station were more about not being able to let go, and that he needed to maintain a link to the atmosphere and the people that had been his 'family' for so long. And of course, for a few months, his every visit was met with smiling, welcoming friendly faces from all of us. He'd come into the office, exchange pleasantries with the duty LA, then wander off down the corridor to the mess room to have a good old chat with the lads. Often from the office I'd hear

'Hey Jack, great to see you. How's Mary?' followed by laughter. This was Jack's tonic; a chance not only to have an hour from his week where he could be back at Henrietta Street, but I was sure that he needed to get out from under Mary's feet too. But as the months went on, Jacks visits became less frequent; still at least once a month though, and as I'd pop round to see him at home he'd say how there were the appearance of new faces who he didn't know, and who didn't know him. Each visit he would see less and less of us and said he felt things were changing. Jack was old school and I knew that change wasn't something he could handle well. I sensed an objection to new staff taking over 'his' station, and a widening gap between him and it. I didn't want to tell him that of course as time goes on more people will leave and change and so compound his problem. One of the old leading ambulancemen of the time, Johnny Richmond retired at a similar time and said that he would never come back to the station. Never would he set foot again in the place that had housed him for 30 years. Not because he hated the place, but because he knew that change would take place and he wouldn't be able to cope with it. I couldn't understand this at the time, but they were wise words and perhaps ones that Jack should have heeded. A couple of years after Jack's retirement, following one of his routine shopping trips, Jack called into station and headed for the office as he always did. But on this day there was no one in the office he knew, but he was met by the smiling face of a relatively new member of staff, Dalziel Wade. Dal was an intellect, and the probable product of a public school education. He was a gentleman, polite but not the best of communicators, but greeted Jack with warmth.

"Good morning sir, can I help you?". A greeting worthy of receipt of a good impression. But Jack was already put out that there were none of his friends in the office. He remained polite but firm.

"I'm Jack. I used to be a leading hand here. I just popped in to say hello to my friends".

"Do you have any identification on you sir", Dal asked "only, I've been instructed to not allow anyone on station who isn't authorised" As far as he was concerned, this was a normal, sensible question, and perhaps to most others it would have appeared so too. But this one comment had a profound effect on Jack and struck deep into his very heart and soul. For it signified to him that Henrietta Street was no longer his; no longer the place where he could come to see his friends. He wasn't welcome here anymore. Struggling to keep his emotion under wraps, Jack replied,

"no son, I don't have any identification on me, but remember this; I was working here for 20 years before you were in nappies, so I don't think I need to prove to you who I am do I?"

Dal often lacked a bit of humanism and common sense, and rather than seeing the situation for what it was, he felt put out by Jack's approach, and reared up.

"you don't need to take that attitude mate, I'm only doing my job. But I guess it'll be alright for a few minutes. There might be someone in the mess room who knows you. I'll show you where it is."

This further angered Jack, and made him feel a real outsider. Staring Dal in the eye, he fired back.

"Like I said son, 30 years on this depot. I think I can find my way to the mess room without your fuckin' help?"

Realising now at this late stage he'd hit a raw nerve, Dal agreed and let him go. And when Jack got to the mess room, there were quite a few people in there. But no one he knew. Henrietta Street station has always had a reputation for being insular towards strangers, including new staff. 'It's our game and you're not playing until we invite you' was the order. But once you get accepted, these people become fiercely loyal comrades. At The Street, a spade was a spade, and if someone had an issue with you, they'd let you know. There's was never any talk behind backs, and never any back stabbing, and over the years, there were a few fights in the mess room, but they always ended with a handshake and a clear atmosphere. I experienced this initial coldness, and now Jack was. But this was one man who shouldn't have. As he stepped into the doorway, the chatter slowed until only one guy taking his snooker shot was left talking, where he hadn't noticed Jack's presence. The 'chink' of the balls stopped and only the voices from the television remained. Jack had been through more than these youngsters could ever have imagined, and he didn't scare easily. But this didn't stop him feeling awkward. Very awkward. The sort of feeling that emphasised that he didn't belong here anymore. It wasn't his, and this turning point was pivotal for Jack. Seeing no one in the mess room he knew, he turned and walked silently back up the corridor, past the open office door and out to the back of the station where his car was still parked. Seeing Jack leaving, Dal called out a cursory 'goodbye sir', to which silence was the reply. Jack was mortified. This was the cut off point. I don't know if he knew it would come one day or if it took him by surprise, but Jack Stowe never set foot in Henrietta Street Ambulance Station again. It was the true end of an era for him that I think he never got over. I continued to call round to see Mary and Jack about twice a year, and still always at Christmas. Every time, Jack would tell me about the incident. Every time. I never thought for a minute that this was dementia or Alzheimers, but it painted a picture of the impact this event had had on him.

The next couple of years saw Jacks physical health decline. He'd been a cigar smoker for all the time I'd known him, and now started getting recurring chest problems and a constant hoarse voice. At the age of 72 Jack sadly passed away. The first I knew about it was getting a phone call from his daughter, who gave me details of the funeral arrangements. Full ambulance service funerals were the domain of staff who died whilst still employed. Jack, of course, had been left for some years by this time and wouldn't qualify for the 'works', but was so highly thought of that management allowed me to take a paramedic motorcycle, and give the hearse an escort to the crematorium. I had left the motorcycle unit by this time but was still big into my bikes, and to say this was an honour for me is a gross injustice. Escorting Jacks final journey allowed me to pay my respects to the great man; the man responsible for changing my life and my direction. This book wouldn't have been written had it not been for him.

On a cold spring morning, the day of the funeral arrived. I'd spent hours cleaning the bike, polishing my leathers and bulling my boots until I could have shaved in them. This level of respect was what this man deserved, and nothing less. The Co Op funeral service conducted the journey in and as we left Jacks house, the street was lined with his neighbours and local friends. I rode in front of the hearse, front blue emergency strobe lights flashing, wearing no fluorescence, only black with a white helmet. It reminded me of Princess Diana's cortège, riding slowly to the crematorium, the bikes presence demonstrating the importance of this man. And upon arrival at the final resting place, the entrance was lined with all Jacks work friends, all those who came to pay their last respects. I'm sure Jack was up there watching, and I wished that all the young people who had seen Jack in the mess room on his last visit could've witnessed how important this man had been; his last visit to the station that had become the turning point that sent him on his decline.

Mary continued to live in the same house after Jacks death but she was never the same. Never again did I see the bubbly innocence, the smile or the happiness. Her eyes became sad and her world had gone, and as so often happens when one half of more than half a century of marriage dies, so too did Mary. She remained with us for a year or two in body, but her soul was always with Jack. Soon she became reunited with her love forever. They're a special couple to me, and are part of my 'butterfly effect', for which I will be eternally grateful.

CHAPTER 2. THE 'NEWBIE'.

Modern day ambulance services in the UK, are run by Chief Executives who answer to The Health Department, and who cascade their desires down through the ranks of the lesser managers until things stop on the 'shop floor' so to speak, with the people who staff the ambulances. Rules and regulations abound, keeping people on their toes and providing full time work for many. Patient treatments are recorded, to the point where on occasion, more time is spent on the paperwork than the initial treatment of the patient. And with the taking on board of the computer allowing for individual, group, area and organisational statistics. Working patterns and clinical delivery are monitored, audited and scrutinised with discrepancies investigated and staff grilled.

But the 1980's saw a very different pattern of work practice. Records were filed in the office on postcards, which were housed in old brown box draws sat on the top of filing cabinets, and where the Leading Ambulanceman, or 'LA', would always put their hand on what they wanted in the blink of an eye. Ambulance cases, or 'jobs', were written up on pink case sheets, with 5 or 6 jobs to one A4 sheet. There was little or no detail of the case as it was given out, aside of the address and what was going on, and following treatment, nothing was recorded as to what had been done for the patient, meaning where staff attended Coroner's Court, good old fashioned memory had to be relied upon, and heaven help you of you couldn't answer a question from The Coroner. Clinical audit didn't really exist, and if you messed up, it was usually discovered because of a complaint from a patient, a family member or your crew mate. Mess room disagreements were still occasionally sorted by aggressive arguments and flying chairs, and if you'd cocked something up, the gaffer or the LA would have you in the office, on your own, and give you one almighty bollocking, and that would be the end of it. You didn't do it again. And you respected the one dishing out the lashing. Remember, I was snotty nosed 21 year old, green behind the ear, whose mother barely knew I was out late at night, up against LA's like Don Jackson, an ex sergeant major of many years whose voice was incredibly low and frightening, even when I hadn't done any wrong. The peak on his cap was vertical, and he walked with his feet turned out slightly and his chest puffed out as his arms swung like he was on a parade ground. You could've shaved in the shine on his boots and his shirts were always immaculately pressed. He reminded me of a cross between Windsor Davies, the Sergeant Major from the 70's sitcom 'It Ain't Half Hot Mum', and Mr Mackay, the fearsome prison officer from another British 70's sitcom, 'Porridge'.

The mess room at Henrietta Street Ambulance Station, despite the buildings demure feel, became quite a welcoming, homely place sometime after I'd settled in. It was a large room with a worn dusty, Parkay floor, big hospital type old fashioned radiators that seemed to be red hot all year round. Big bore, exposed, above floor pipes fed these radiators, increasing the room temperature even more and necessitating the opening of the windows wide even in the freezing winters. A grand full sized snooker table adorned the one end of the room with plentiful space surrounding it to play. The Eagles social club, so called because the station's radio call sign was 'Eagle', was particularly proud of this table and tournaments were a regular feature of the social calendar. It was re-covered regularly, and cosseted by many. Around the edge of two sides of the room were about 25 easy chairs, placed side by side for the length of the walls; wooden framed with brown, vinyl covered foam squabs and backs, and which were surprisingly comfortable. Separating the mess room from the kitchen was a servery with hatch. The kitchen was well laid out in true catering style with stainless steel and white tiles everywhere, with a big water boiler being the centre piece on the far wall. In between the snooker table and the servery sat a table and chairs, enough to accommodate 14 or 15 people.

The ambulance service was very militaristic at these times, and indeed many of the old hands had served in the forces and still kept their culture going in this environment. They didn't take well to new boys, especially 21 year olds, despite my approach of knowing nothing, and not being afraid to let others know it. Henrietta Street had a gruesome reputation among other stations for being arrogant and unwelcoming, so following my initial training course, arriving as the new boy into a 'clicky' environment, was a daunting task. On my first morning out, I duly reported to the Station Office, where Jack met me and took me down to the mess room. His was to be the only welcoming face that cold morning. The front line shift had only just come on at 7 o'clock that morning, but I was working on the outpatients and wouldn't start until eight.

The outpatient drivers were deemed the lowest of the low; they were the broom sweepers of the service, and I was happy to accept my place. I saw the front line guys as Gods. They were life savers, so knowledgeable and important. Little did I realise at that stage, that most of them didn't have much theoretical knowledge. It was being street wise and experienced that made them successful; knowing when someone was really sick and on death's door just because....well, they knew. It was a total mystery to me then how they did it, but they did. Many of them couldn't have told you much about pressure gradients or quoted gas laws, but they fixed broken limbs, stopped bleeding and delivered babies using this experience and heaps of common sense. Many of them had joined the service needing little more than a driving licence and completed only a basic first aid course when they'd started many years before.

Jack led me down the corridor and showed me the door to the mess room, inside of which there was a fair bit of noise going on, with male voices, the TV and the occasional female laughter. I turned to Jack for some moral support or an introduction as I now stood in the doorway. But he was turning the corner into the office at the other end of the corridor. I gulped hard and walked forward. Two blokes were playing snooker; the one taking the shot concentrating hard. The other leaned on his cue and diverted his gaze from the impending sinking of the yellow, to me. I looked at him expecting compassion but was quickly disappointed, as his mate said something I didn't catch and the two of them laughed. Around the main table sat several people who ignored me as they read their papers or played scrabble, and in the middle of the row of more comfortable chairs was a woman in her forties, I'd have guessed, laughing with a big fat bloke. She was a dark haired woman with a round jolly face, clearly enjoying a banter. I caught the tail end of the story.

"…………well, I just knew I was goin' to shit meself."

She moved her legs like a sumo wrestler in front of his opponent. She continued, now breaking into a raucous laugh so she could hardly finish the sentence. Something else was said and the two of them flung their heads back roaring, the tears clearly visible on her face. The blokes at the table never stirred. Then the snooker player piped up.

"Val, you never fail to amaze."

"Well, I couldn't help it could I?" She replied, "it was those bleeding pies I'd had from the cafe. He's a dirty bastard he is. Never washes 'is 'ands after e's 'ad a shit".

The laughing continued. And at least for the next few seconds, the focus had diverted from me. But now I had to walk forwards into this foreboding place; the lions den. I spotted a comfy chair in the corner, away from anyone else, where I could go and hide, and wait my time out until 8 o'clock. I crept past the boys at the table and approached the chair.

"Don't think you're gonna sit there sonny. That's Arthur's seat".

My back was to them and I didn't know who'd spoken. The focus was back on me, and I could feel my cheeks becoming hotter.

"Oh, sorry", I said, now feeling really uncomfortable.

"Nor the one next to it. That's George's. You're over there, in the other corner." The voice continued. I felt like the 'other' corner was where murderers and rapists were sent to.

Then the lady spoke up,

"Oh let him sit down Rod. Anyway, B shift ain' even on. Arthurs just finished nights"

The disturbing voice belonged to another fat bloke with a beard and aged about 50.

"So fuckin' what? He shouldn't be sittin' 'ere anyway. E's on the granny runs".

I was quite happy to leave the room at that point; to get out of the firing line, and seek sanctuary elsewhere, and seriously considered walking out on the pre-tense of using the toilet, but that would be cowardly. So I diligently sat where I was told and before too long a fresh faced girl came bouncing in, walking past all the front liners without a word said and approached me. She was about 30 with short hair and average looks, but with a brightness about her. And definitely my saviour.

"You must be Dave. I'm Elaine".

DAVID BRADBURY

She made everything better, just in that one sentence. That one smile.

CHAPTER 3. A STEEP LEARNING CURVE.

In the first few months, working on the outpatient sector of the service, seemed to a keen, motivated 21 year old to be boring and pointless. Picking up the elderly and infirm and driving them to their day centre and out patient appointments, then home afterwards. There was no action, and the work was repetitive, and I longed for not knowing where I would be in five minutes time. I craved to work shifts and wanted to be immersed in this exciting world of blood, guts and gore. I did however, settle in and calmed down when it was obvious that despite previous outpatient drivers getting a 'six week course', the one needed to progress up to front line, in a matter of a few months, money was tight and no courses would be forthcoming for the foreseeable future. I look back now at the young, inexperienced man I was then. I never realised that this time spent on the 'granny runs', was invaluable and incredibly important. It was my apprenticeship, and formed the foundation of such skills as manual handling, driving, geography of Birmingham and topography of the community I was to go on and serve. Perhaps the biggest skill learned and honed, and it is a skill, was communication. Later on in my career, when teaching pre hospital care, I would be regularly saying to new recruits that the job of caring for the community in the prehospital field is 10% knowledge, 40% common sense and 50% communication. And if you don't develop it, it's a destiny for failure. Having the gift of the gab, and of listening, has almost certainly saved my hide in one way or another on more occasions than I care to mention.

It was November 1987 and I'd taken up the opportunity at Jack's suggestion, to go out as an observer with the emergency crews after my own day work was done. His advice was simple. If I wanted to be accepted, always ask to go out with them and never assume, clean the front line trucks and make the tea. A sure fire guarantee of success.

Settling well into life on the outpatient sector saw weekdays go by with a slow but enjoyable pace. Slow, because like the childish look forward to Christmas morning and all the excitement the presents bring, so the end of the week heralded going out with the emergency crews, and the immersion into the world of blood, guts and gore I so desired.

Early evening Friday saw peace and quiet in the mess room at Henrietta Street, which continued for some time. The low hum of the television making up the background, along with the occasional 'chink' of the snooker balls from the table. The air above the room had the customary haze of cigar smoke and the atmosphere was one of relaxed anticipation for me. I snoozed in the easy chair when the red emergency phone rang and broke the silence. Most of the blokes remained quiet and still and I wondered who would come forward to answer it. Then a cheery Laurie came skipping up the corridor and picked up the phone with an enthusiastic tone.

"Hello, Henrietta Street dog's home," he said. There was a long pause before he acknowledged the caller, thanked them and put the put the phone down before telling them which crew was going on this job. I knew Laurie a little, as a friendly bloke who worked with Kelly Peterson and together were known as a pair of comedians. I'd been out with them a couple of times and related to their humour. Their classic style, when entering a traffic roundabout on a job, was to ask me to fetch a first aid bag from the rear cupboard of the ambulance. Of course I'd oblige, standing up just as the vehicle lurched hard right throwing me all over the back of the ambulance. Much to all our amusement.

Back in the mess room, Laurie turned to me.

"You wanna come young 'un? We got a stabbing. You might learn something."

In the blink of an eye my adrenaline levels shot through the roof, as I stood up trying to give the impression of a relaxed nonchalant individual, failing dismally.

"Yeah, OK……er, if thats alright with you guys." I replied in Laurie's direction, but he was already half out of the room legging it to the garage where our awaiting ambulance sat. Kelly was already in the garage working on his car, as was the norm in those days.

We all jumped in Eagle 3, and with sliding doors still open and no time for the placement of seatbelts, off we shot at breakneck speed. The story was that someone had been stabbed in a pub around the corner from the hospital. Little else was known. These were the days when actions needed to be less accountable than of present, and so the speeds and manner of driving, by modern standards, left much to be desired. Blue emergency beacons flashed and two-tone air horns screamed to get drivers out of the way, and with two stretchers in the rear saloon of the vehicle, and little else, this was cutting edge technology. The powerful engine covered the three or four miles in a matter of minutes, and even though I had been thrown around in the back of the ambulance like a rag doll, we arrived on scene and out we all jumped to be met by mayhem. There were shouts and screams from panicking people trying to get us into the patient as quickly as possible. This was my first real taste of a panicking crowd and one I'd be seeing many, many more time over the next four decades. Experience however has led me to realise that actually there is often little correlation between the degree of anxiety and excitement from onlookers and the level of severity of the patient. Often the calm onlooker will be hiding a deceased individual and vice versa. Here, a crowd of excited people had gathered on the street and directed us into the pub where it transpired a fight had broken out some 15 minutes prior and as a result someone had been stabbed.

I followed Kelly in, and we were ushered in to the bar, a vinyl floored room full of cigarette smoke and a one arm bandit. The smell of stale alcohol mixed with excitement, and as we entered, the crowds parted and there before us was a man lying on his back, in a large pool of claret, motionless with a blood soaked shirt and his eyes half closed. There was a strange smell in the air and one I would learn to recognise. It hinted at a metallic, iron like odour. Subsequent experience would tell me it was blood, and if it could be smelt, there was a lot of it.

Even with my level of inexperience, I could tell he was in a serious condition. Kelly got to work while Laurie went back outside to get some gear. The patient's shirt was ripped off and a large dressing was applied to a stab wound to his chest. It was an open, gaping split with blood oozing out. Once in place Kelly checked for a pulse, and not finding one, he started CPR and chest compressions. He looked at me with a certain degree of stern concentration.

"Dave, start chest compressions while I try and stop the bleeding."

I didn't have time to contemplate and did as I was instructed while preparations were made to get the poor patient loaded onto the carry chair to be whisked quickly to the ambulance. Laurie had already pre alerted the hospital of our arrival because it was literally 15 seconds drive and there wouldn't be time to get them ready for our arrival once we set out.

Before I knew it the patient was loaded onto the back of the ambulance for the drive to Dudley Road Hospital casualty dept.

These were the very early days of paramedic care and where this crew had a realisation that this patient needed to be on the surgeons table and that no amount of prehospital care would save him. So we were met with a flurry of medical bodies in the hospital, the doctors of which decided that this patient needed an open thoracotomy and so before my very eyes they cracked his chest open and did what they had to. Laurie decided I needed to get a better look and so grabbed me from the outside onlookers and shoved me next to the doctor.

It was hard for me to contemplate exactly what I was seeing in my extreme inexperience. The equipment - a mixture of barbaric devices designed to crack open the chest, scalpels, drapes, probes, and spikes, with a health mix of finger manually plugging up holes in the heart caused by the knife. This was certainly a baptism of fire for this young, wet behind the ear ambulance trainee.

The excitement carried on for a short while until the doctors decided it was fruitless and that this poor individual had indeed dropped off the perch. His time was up, and resuscitative measures ceased. My emotions ran high. There before lay a naked male, with his chest butchered open, tubes sticking everywhere, more blood that I'd ever seen decorating the patient, the floor and those who been in contact with him, including me. It was plastered over my hands, arms, shirt and pretty much the rest of my uniform.

My head was still spinning from what was to the first serious case of many now under my belt. We returned to station to clean up. When this involved the removal of the stretchers and the use of a high pressure hose on the vehicle wash with the doors open, ceiling, sides and floor, it would signal the sheer amount of blood which decorated the inside. Diluted rivers of

DAVID BRADBURY

it ran down the drain. Then the cursory cup of tea and natural debrief between us allowed the truck to dry and be prepared for the next case.

CHAPTER 4. THE EARLY DAYS.

Shortly after serving my first couple of months at Henrietta Street Ambulance Station, I was moved to Sutton Coldfield Ambulance Station, to work on The Good Hope Hospital Day Centre run. Sutton had a beckoning appeal about it. Somehow friendlier than Henrietta Street, it had an air that I'd actually achieved something by being sent there, almost like a promotion. And it had its fair share of characters too. One of the more notable was John Berke. A short chap who wore his cap pushed back on his head and always smoked a pipe which was welded to his bottom lip, so he resembled Popeye. And as this was before the days of banned smoking, John lit up anywhere and anytime; the mess room, the hospital, and when picking up patients. A veteran of some 30 years, he was coasting for retirement and now worked with the out patients as I did, but his experience meant whereas I struggled with some aspects of the job, he made it seem all too easy. And he became a great mentor, having a wonderful bedside manner with the patients, and a great supportive approach to us young 'uns. That is towards all but Troy Showett. Troy had started life some years earlier on front line at Henrietta Street, but for whatever reason, had opted to come off and work on out patients, being moved to Sutton. There was a side to him which some found annoying, and which I never really understood, but he was a gentle man who never seemed to get wound up by anybody and refused to go along with the regime of jokes and micky taking, and perhaps it was this that made him a target for John whose antics showed not one hint of mercy and worsened as the time went on. Troy took a pride in polishing his boots every morning when he came in, but every morning, John would hide the shoe polish to try to get Troy annoyed. But Troy would calmly search for it until he found it, angering John all the more, who then took to replacing the polish with a mixture of black shoe polish and lard. But still Troy wouldn't react. His coffee mug would disappear; he'd bring in another. His peaked cap would go missing; he'd go without. His moped would be roped up into the rafters of the garage, and if he couldn't retrieve it, he'd walk home without complaint. The bullying was relentless, but still Troy wouldn't react, and neither would he complain, although this was an era of this sort of behaviour and probably would have fallen on deaf ears anyway.

Although the very bottom rung of the ladder, I quite enjoyed these times even though I hampered after the more exciting work. I lived in Sutton, and it was much easier to get to by commute, and now involved a split shift; 0800hrs to 1200, then 1400 to 1800. A nice long lunch break, but I'd rather have finished work earlier. The vehicle I worked on fetched the 'clientele' for the day centre in the morning, taking them home in the afternoon. Some came several days a week, and some only once, and they consisted of mainly mild dementia or mobility issue elderly ladies and gents who were able to live in the community with family or sometimes on their own, with the support of the day centre who gave them a hot meal and some mental stimulation through occupational therapy. It got them out of the house, and kept them going.

I started working with Karen Benjamin. We manned the ambulance which picked up all the 'two man lifts', that is, all those that couldn't walk unaided, or at all and who needed assistance from the two of us. There was also a solo vehicle running from Sutton. This one-manned vehicle serviced the day centre at Highcroft Psychiatric hospital, where 99% of the patients were able to walk well. Not long after I started, Dave Flore came to Sutton, and he and Karen were crewed up allowing me to have a taste of solo work which I really enjoyed. It afforded me the opportunity to go where I wanted, when I wanted so long as I picked up the right people in the morning and dropped them off after lunch. This solo working pattern was to form the basis of most of my career, proceeding shortly after qualifying as a paramedic onto the Motorcycle Unit, then later as a solo officer, and more recently as a single officer in Queensland's central outback.

Dave was a tall, skinny guy of my age, with a wispy tach and sharp features. He loved his beer and smoked heavily, often being found in The Trout and Mullet on a Friday and Saturday evening and again over Sunday lunch. We immediately hit it off, with a similar frustration at wanting to get on front line. Our sense of living the moment and humour also matched. But Dave hated working with Karen. Their personalities just didn't gel, and Dave had a short fuse for intolerance of people he didn't get on with. I, on the other hand, found her OK, but for some reason, he just couldn't abide her, and began to avoid working with her at all costs. Eventually he pleaded with me to work with him permanently and let Karen do the solo work. I loved the walking cases but Dave was persuasive and reluctantly, I agreed. And so started our friendship.

One of the good elements of working the day centres, was getting to know the ladies and gents we picked up very well. After all, we saw some of them every day, and with some we built up a great rapport. And they loved us. The 'two Daves', we became known as, 'little Dave' and 'big Dave'; and how they plied us with cakes, chocolate, drinks and sweets. It's alleged, that we made more in Christmas tips than we actually earned for that week. But we denied everything as being gossip. And never a day, nor barely a patient went by when we didn't have a laugh, or a joke with them. Many said that they hated the day centre, finding it condescending and boring, and that the only reason they continued coming was because they looked forward to seeing the 'two Daves'.

One such lady was Florence Gertrude Pearson, or Flo as she was affectionately known. We had a fondness for her, which saw us give her names of Dirty Gerty from number 30, or Flying Flo, always used with compassion for someone we came to love. Flo had succumbed to a stroke some years before and lived with her husband Norm, in sheltered accommodation at the top end of Birmingham. Norm regarded himself as a bit of a lady's man but we always saw him as a little harsh, and who always gave the impression that he resented her disability. We suspected that he didn't always treat her with the respect she deserved, but was always pleasant to her in our company. Flo was always happy, and had an incredible outlook on life. No youngster, and at the age of about 75, she was confined to a wheelchair and wasn't able to speak, But she could laugh, and smile, and loved the banter we gave her, as we moved her from wheelchair to the ambulance seating. One of us would get in close to her with our arms around her, lifting and shifting her on the count of three.

"Come on Flo, give yer toy boy a big hug. But no tongues mind, or I'll tell Norm." Or

"Ooo Flo, you mind where you're putting your hands when we have hugs like this. My missus'll be getting jealous!"

She'd start laughing, and often used to break wind as she did. So much so, that Flo's farting became legendary. On a good day she was able to weight bare, not walk mind, but she could stand allowing an easier transition from chair to chair. In these circumstances Dave and I would get either side of her whilst she was seated in her wheelchair, under each arm, and with a "one, two, three", we would lift her into the standing position. We discovered though, that as she bore down to try to stand, this was when her wind was most fruitful, and by varying the amount we assisted at any given moment, she would increase or decrease the amount she bore down. Thus, Dave and I could play tunes on Flo's wind. Much to Flo's amusement. One day she laughed so much she wee'd herself. But then so very nearly did Dave and I.

Then, as happens with people as precious as these, Flo died. Norm had found her one Saturday morning, cold and lifeless, and had called an emergency ambulance. She'd passed peacefully in her sleep. The same emergency crew were on duty on the Monday morning, and knowing we normally picked her up, Phil said to me,

"Dave, you pick up Florence Pearson don't ya?"

"Yeah", I replied, "why?"

"Well you needn't bother again, she croaked it on Sat'dy morning".

It didn't really strike me as surprising, but his nonchalant tone, the way he cast aside this lady who I held in as high an esteem as my own grandmother, annoyed me. I didn't say anything to him about the way he said it; it wasn't the done thing. Besides, I was trying to get in with the lads on front line to get them to take me out. But it didn't stop me feeling upset inside. Flo was gone. The smiles, the laughs, the chat, the person. But she'd be replaced by others who'd be different, but equally as nice, who'd make my working days that bit more special.

CHAPTER 5. FATES' CHANGE OF PLANS.

For several months prior, Dave and Karen worked crewed up servicing the Good Hope Day Hospital. I was put onto the Highcroft run. Highcroft was the local psychiatric hospital which had a day centre called Treeview being for walking cases only, so I worked on my own, this suiting me well, and giving me the taste of solo working that was to last for some time. Highcroft Hospital was a former Poor Law institution, before becoming a psychiatric hospital, and there was a social stigma to being treated there. The original Highcroft Hall was built between 1869 and 1871 by Victorian architect, Yeoville Thomason and the original building was sanctioned by the Poor Law Board as a workhouse providing housing to paupers, idiots, tramps, seniles, lunatics and imbeciles (terms used at the time with distinctive definitions).

The building was originally named the Aston Union Workhouse although it was renamed over the years to Erdington House (1912 - following the City boundary changes), Highcroft Hall Hospital (1942) and was more commonly referred to in later years as just Highcroft Hospital. Over the years, the hospital had generally provided care for the mentally ill. In 1994, it became part of the Northern Birmingham Mental Health NHS Trust, and during the following two years, the facilities were gradually rehoused in more modern units nearby. In 1996, the building was declared closed.

The site was derelict for the subsequent eight years, before being refurbished by property developers in 2004-2006.

In 1988, when I was serving Treeview, the hospital itself was very much as it had been for decades before. Driving through the large, depressing, brick archway entrance, the three storey hospital loomed out in front like a prisoner of war camp. There was nothing bright about the place; no flowers, few trees, and it gave the typical stereotype image of a lunatic asylum. The brick shell had drab, smog stained walls, with sash windows sitting on large grey sills. Some had bars, but all had the same gloomy appearance, and the same story to tell of what each had seen in the rooms they looked into; the sort of place I only ever imagined when the weather was equally grey and depressing, and it was hard for my mind's eye to picture it in the warm sunshine of summer. Walking through the heavy wooden doors, the inside had long corridors, big radiators and an echoing spooky feel about the place. You could almost hear screaming and moaning from some poor soul shut up in a locked, barred cell, and I often imagined, that around the next corner I would meet an inmate, dressed in a long, dirty white robe, oblivious to me, looking into space as she walked, chanting and laughing with insanity. But of course, this was just the over imagination of a 22 year old. The reality was that the place was staffed by a team of caring nurses where the patients were treated with the respect and compassion they deserved, no where better demonstrated than the day centre, which had been created only a few years before to cater for the Erdington and Sutton Coldfield population who were generally older and having the more mature psychiatric issues of dementia or Alzheimer's disease.

Tony attended the day centre Monday through Friday, and I first met him when I was driving the walking cases into the day centre. A dapper man with a neat, impeccably trimmed moustache, he always wore a shirt and tie with casual trousers, and I imagined him gardening, servicing his car or decorating the house wearing the same attire. He was from the Brylcreme era and always smelled pleasantly with his hair neat and his shoes polished. A none smoker, he appeared a very fit man physically, of medium height and build and was only 58, putting him somewhat younger than my average passenger. Tony was initially a little quiet, almost introverted, but would speak when spoken to and was polite and gentle. As the first week progressed, I became acquainted with Wendy, who I assumed was his daughter, who would send him off in the morning and greet him back in the afternoon, like a child going to and from school. She'd remind him to ask Angie the nurse when he wanted the toilet at the day centre, and to eat all his dinner, to which he would turn his head roughly in her direction without uttering anything. She'd pack him off with a kiss on the cheek, referring to him as 'love', to which he never responded, almost like she hadn't done it. He reminded me of the educationally subnormal individual who does as they are told, and doing little until they are told to do so.

As the days and weeks progressed, I noticed Tony changing. In the first few days he walked upright, like a man on a mission. Although not tall, he stood erect with his head up and his face bright, even though he said little. By the third week, his stance had changed to that of fragility. He became hunched over, looking at the ground as he walked, like the hunchback man, his pace slowed and steps shortened to that of someone with Parkinson's disease. This has a very specific trait in the way they walk. Steps taken are very small with a shuffle of step, occasionally stumbling and hesitating with the next step as if the foot knows what it wants to do but isn't quite sure how to get there.

Tony worsened as the days went on. His appearance changed. One Tuesday morning, he shuffled out of the house unshaven, with a couple of days of stubble and remnants of his breakfast stuck to his chin, and finely coating his shirt. His tie was missing and his shirt's buttons were out of sink with the holes they went into by one, giving a distorted look to his upper half. The sleeves were ruffled and the wrist buttons loose, with only part of the shirt tucked into a pair of dirty trousers that were visibly several sizes too big for his waist, and in fear of falling down. Looking down at Tony's feet as he shuffled near to my bus, I noted his feet were socked but lacked shoes. He looked like a poor demented man of 80, and quite pathetic. His demeanour was the same though; hunched over and oblivious to anything and everything. There was no kiss from Wendy on this morning. She stood at the doorway, visibly upset and crying as Tony had walked past her. She watched him as he neared me, giving a half hearted wave in my direction as she became aware of me looking at her, before disappearing back inside and shutting the door gently. I could see through the glass pane she stood behind, as she remained there, that the crying continued. Her head sunk into her hands as it bobbed with grief. I stood by the side of the ambulance to assist Tony up the step and into his seat. I caught the strong smell of faeces as I held his arm and hand, and was glad we had plastic seats in the bus; it would make for easier cleaning later.

As the weeks had gone on, it was almost measurable, almost predictable, that the next time I would see Tony, he would be worse. But I wasn't prepared for this. It had only been the weekend and a bank holiday Monday, three days, since I'd seen him. A decline in his walk, his stance, his concentration, his communication, his everything. It got me to thinking, that if his decline was this quick, it probably wasn't that long ago that he was 'normal'. I thought about asking his daughter, but decided it was cheeky, nosey, and not my place to know. I was merely his driver; the one who took him to rest-bite care every day. It wasn't my place to ask. I was a nobody. But, being human, I had a curiosity that had to be satisfied. I'd built up a good friendly relationship with Wendy over the weeks. I usually went to the front door to collect him, and dropped him back off at the same point upon our return, having a bit of a chat with her each time, of how the weather was, and how her father had got on that day, and what he'd been up to.

I'd always assumed that the house where Tony was living was his daughter's. It was a nice, albeit small, terraced dwelling in a quiet, short cul-de-sac in Walmley, Sutton Coldfield, and was the nearest of my pickups, and drop offs to Sutton Ambulance Station, and so was the last drop off of the day. The day centre had cleaned Tony up when I went to collect him for the home bound journey. He had a different set of clothes on, still not his size, but at least they were clean, properly fastened, and he was now wearing a pair of white training type shoes, which mismatched perfectly with the brown trousers he had on. He was now clean shaven and smelt somewhat fresher. I had earlier had words with Mary, one of the Treeview staff of my concerns, and had the reassuring reply that she would take good care of him and clean him up. So, on that Tuesday afternoon of week four with nobody left on the ambulance waiting, I arrived at Wendy's house, pulling up at the driveway, and jumping out to go round to assist Tony off the bus. But the normally quiet Tony didn't jump up as he normally did. This time he appeared drowsy and was more slumped in his seat. I encouraged him to stand up which he eventually did, before he began the long and arduous trek to get off the vehicle and walk the 10 yards to the front door. The normal one minute, now took five, and getting him down the steps off the ambulance was difficult, and at one point I thought I would need help. But we managed. Tony's decline was now so painfully obvious. Wendy hurried towards us as we approached her on the driveway, and with one of us under each arm, we gently helped Tony inside the house where we continued into the lounge, sitting him in an upright armchair. He sat down without protest, and almost immediately changed from his trance like state to that of sleep, his bottom jaw dropping, eyes closing, and a gentle snore starting. Wendy thanked me for my help and asked if I would like a cup of tea. This was the perfect opportunity to glean the information I had so wondered about.

Wendy was a lady of about 40, I'd guessed. She had a semi smart appearance, and gave me the impression she was a secretary or a receptionist.

"Milk and sugar?" She asked

"Yes. Please. Both" I replied, thankful the conversation had restarted after a few minutes silence had ensued, while the tea making process was underway.

"Wendy?", I started with a little hesitation. "Pardon me if I appear nosy, but what's your dad diagnosed with?

"Dad?" She whipped around starring me in the eye with a harsh look on her face for a few long seconds, before her brow sank, her face lightened, and a wry smile appeared.

"Tony's my....well my....sort of husband. We've been together for these last fifteen years. We were going to marry, but never got round to it."

I was so embarrassed, and felt my cheeks glowing. I stuttered and stumbled out a barrage of words and apologies.

"Oh don't worry," she reassured with a comforting tone. "Tony's 18 years older than me. Huh, a few months go, looking at him, you'd never have known though. D'ya know, he had thick black hair, and a body that women craved for. He dressed classy like, and wore expensive after shave. Now look at him", she said as her tone faded and she stared at the ground. "These last few months have taken their toll. On both of us".

This was the time I wanted the hole to open up and swallow me, and was the first of two occasions which taught me a very good lesson. There is a saying in the ambulance service, probably coined by me, which says 'assumption is the mother of all fuck ups'. The second occasion which sealed my learning experience, was a year or two later, (yes, you'd have thought I'd have learned by now) when speaking to a young lady in her early 20's, of medium build, with a large protrusion from her abdomen, and I'd guessed was about 7 or 8 months pregnant, sat next to an older woman with grey hair aged in her 40's. They were in a women's hostel.

"Sooooo", I started towards the older woman."Looking forward to becoming a granny?" I said, with a beaming smile on my face. She glared at me, with a dagger drawn.

"A granny? What ya mean?"

"Well, you know, when the baby's born." I pointed to the belly of the woman sat next to her, whose face was now pointed angrily in my direction.

"I'm not her mother, she's my sister!"

Where's that bloody hole, I need again?' Rang through my head. Bad enough? Well, no actually, because then the younger lady, having computed what I'd said, then piped up,

"And I ain't pregnant! You sayin' I'm fat?"
Like I say, 'assumption is the mother of all..........'

I digress. My embarrassment with Wendy was short lived. She could see I'd meant no offence and was used to others thinking the same. After all, an age gap of nearly 20 years between partners is unusual. She reassured me, as she handed the steaming mug over, which I accepted with pursed lips, as my eyes went embarrassingly still, from Wendy, to the floor. Then the conversation resumed. It didn't seem right to talk in front of Tony, so we naturally stayed in the kitchen. And even though I doubted whether Tony was still awake, or even that he'd comprehend what was going to be said, Wendy pushed the kitchen door to, as she beckoned me to sit at the table. I heard

Tony's soft snore get quieter as the door closed.

Over the next half an hour, Wendy explained what the situation was.

Tony and Wendy had their own printing business, which they'd started some years before. And they'd worked hard to build it up to become quite profitable. Tony was the marketing brains behind it, and spent most of his time on the road, visiting customers. Wendy ran the shop floor, with what sounded like a firm hand. They had several people working for them and as the years passed they enjoyed the high life, holidaying abroad in their Spanish apartment, running two expensive cars, and living in a five bedroomed house in the better part of town. Tony was suave and handsome and his looks belied his mature years. He dressed with, and smelled of, Armani, and took a real pride in his appearance. Tony had always worked on the principle that he was the business's shop window. If he looked good, his customers had confidence in him. Their profits, by the sound of it, bore him out. And he kept himself fit too, running several times a week, and had competed in local marathons several times.

Then some 8 months before, things started going wrong. Wendy noticed him becoming moody and agitated, where his norm was bright and happy. She thought the stress was getting to him and they went to Spain for a couple of weeks. But, she'd stated, he was worse, and the holiday had been a complete nightmare. Tony had even gotten himself into a fight at a bar, something, which for a man of his gentle nature, just couldn't happen. Wendy still thought it was stress related and managed to persuade him to go and see their GP when they returned. He was prescribed anti depressants which worsened things dramatically. The business was suffering and they were losing customers. But that wasn't what worried Wendy so much. Tony's moods abated but he started acting strangely. No longer would he dress smartly, preferring to sit in the chair for long periods apparently starring into space. Then one day, when Wendy came home, she found Tony eating a tin of cat food from the fridge. The house had been rearranged; ornaments had been moved from the mantelpiece to the stairs, chairs were strategically turned upside down and piled upon each other and there was cutlery placed across the hall floor. Wendy didn't know how to deal with this and called her friend, a nurse, who in turn arranged for the doctors to section Tony, that is take him into hospital even against his will.

This was a trying time, Wendy had said. The business went down hill, and they laid off all the staff. The payments on the cars and the mortgage stopped and they were repossessed, forcing her to move into the small rented town house that I knew. Tony was moved to a psychiatric hospital and was diagnosed with early dementia. Wendy had him out as soon as his medication had stabilised him. But the doctors had warned her that Tonys demise would be rapid, due to the type of condition he had. His medication was not meant to cure him; it was palliative care designed to sedate him and make him manageable. But I had seen the ferocity of speed of his decline. Wendy had described, that on that morning, Tony remained in the same clothes he'd been in all weekend, not having visited the toilet once, but just doing it in his trousers and not caring, or not being able to care about sitting in his own mess. He'd been violent all the weekend, not allowing Wendy near him. And on that morning, as she'd approached him, he'd struck her across the face. He might have lost his awareness, and some considerable weight, but the mark bore the evidence of a punch dealt with some force. Wendy clearly felt helpless. She was forced to accept their situation and demise, and her demeanour showed that she wasn't hopeful for the future. And on her behalf, neither was I.

With my cup now empty, I thanked Wendy and left, walking past Tony in his state-lent institutional chair, with easy wipe down sides. His back arched; his chin on his chest, complete with a few days growth of silvered stubble, and brown liquid seeping from the corner of his mouth and stringing onto his shirt. His soft snoring still apparent. He had become a pathetic, senile old man, trapped in what had been the body of a young fit man. His dreams of a long retirement in Spain, gone in almost an instant.

The following morning, I turned up at Tony and Wendy's house as usual, but there was no answer to repeated knocking. I called it through to my controller via my vehicle radio. They asked me to wait one, while they checked. A couple of minutes later they came back to say that the journey had been cancelled and to carry on, which I did, wandering what the issue was. I collected my other ladies and gents and upon arrival at Treeview, Angie informed me that Tony had been admitted to Good Hope Hospital Emergency Dept late in the previous evening. For what, she didn't know, but following informing me, she carried on with the other patients like Tony hadn't meant anything to her. And maybe he hadn't. But he had to me.

I never saw Tony again. And never found out his fate. All I know is that he never came to Treeview again, and I presume that he withered and died shortly after I last saw him. Life is precious and fate can deliver a harsh blow. Is there any difference between the young, fit, healthy 20 year old, full of life and with a promising future whose evening out ends in the fatal and tragic car accident.....and Tony's story?

How fragile is life?

CHAPTER 6. THE TRAGIC TALE OF A LADY.

Many of the 'clientele' of Treeview were characters; individuals who had traits that set them apart from others and made them special in one way or another. Louber Petrovinski was one such person. A tall, thick set man of about 60, with a big, handlebar moustache that reminded me of the turn of the 20th century weight lifters in their black leotards. He was always rough shaven with several days growth and few, if any, teeth, so his bottom jaw protruded beyond his top, like the proverbial gurning man. He walked with the same posture and tone of many chronic, institutionalised, psychiatric patients of the era; a slow, slouched, hunched over, almost Parkinsonian style, looking constantly at the ground. He sported a number 4 crew cut and chain smoked, so constantly had a cigarette hanging out of his mouth or perched between the fingers of his hand. Consequently, his moustache and fingers were stained dark brown. And he wore the same suit jacket; light grey over a dirty pale tee shirt, with un-matching trousers.

Lou lived in totally supported housing; a normal house owned by the state in which lived several residents who would normally have resided in the same psychiatric hospital where most of them went to the day hospital. Apparently it was cheaper and designed to integrate these residents back into society, decisions made by people in their ivory towers, in my opinion, who had little idea of the ideals they were working towards. Lou would never lead a 'normal' life in society. He was too institutionalised. Left to his own devices, Lou would do nothing. His meals were prepared for him, his clothes laid out, his shoe laces tied and he was told when to go out, when to wash, and when to go to bed. And because his living conditions were designed to try and integrate him back, less was done for him as time went on to encourage him to do more for himself. But it wasn't working and was clear as time went on that Lou began to smell of body odour, his clothes were dirty and his stubble got longer. It was obvious to all that he wasn't doing as the ivory towers presumed he would.

With his medication, Lou generally did as he was told, occasionally going off the rails and ending up being admitted back into hospital for several months where they would medicate him, stabilise him, and I would see him back in my ambulance every morning again. Lou was absolutely obsessed with all things sexual, and I always imagined that in his days before psychiatric issue, he was some kind of porn star, having women whenever he wanted them, and creating a reputation of some kind of sexual Adonis. Aside of knowing that he originated from Poland, I knew little of his past, but the reality is that he probably came over some years before as a road worker or labourer, already inbuilt with psychiatric and sexual issues, got caught up with crime and following having served his time, he came to the attention of the Mental Health teams.

If he sat next to any of the women, he would often try and touch them up or suggest they had sex with him. His English was extremely limited with his vocabulary consisting of 'oh yeah sex, yeah', 'fuck' and 'Margareeeet'. In the couple of years I knew Lou, I don't honestly remember him saying anything else. He liked Margaret, a grossly obese, chain smoking and gentle lady, who was another resident from the sheltered house he lived in. She also travelled to Treeview daily with Lou, and knew not to sit next to him on the ambulance. Sometimes if she got on first, he would sit next to her, and in the one mile it took to get to the day centre, I would hear an emulation from the rear of the vehicle.

"Stop it Lou", keep yer 'ands to yerself, yer dirty bastud".

This was rapidly followed by me looking in the mirror and reinforcing Margaret's words to Lou, to get him to stop feeling her leg. But despite his approach, he wasn't a sexual predator. I mean, I never factually knew what his past held, but despite his talk, his actions were little more than a perverted touch up, and it was only ever aimed at Margaret, who was far from the stereo-typical 'attractive' woman. But I appreciate that beauty is in the eye of the beholder.

Another character was Enid Preston. Enid was an elderly but agile lady of 90 years, in 1988, who lived in a local home for the elderly mentally infirm. It was situated about 500 yards from the entrance to Highcroft Hospital. Again, as with the others, I'd draw up along side the entrance to where she lived, beep the horn at between 0830 and 0845, and out would trot Enid, immediately upon hearing the horn, with her coat on and clutching her big brown handbag. Enid was a creature of habit and did everything by time, doing the same things every day, at exactly the same time. Every morning she would be woken at 7 am, be washed, dressed and down at the breakfast table by 7.30. Having eaten always the same thing of half a piece of toast and a cup of tea, she would have her coat put on and would be sat in the hallway to wait the three quarters of an hour before I would arrive. And there she would sit, watching the world go by, with her coat on, clutching her bag, waiting for me.

My initial impression of Enid was that she was a miserable old woman. She never spoke a word in all the time I knew her, not one word, despite me always speaking to her with compassion.

"Morning Enid, have a good weekend?" Or at pickup time from the day centre to go home. "What sort of a day have you had Enid?"

Only to be ignored as she would walk past me without even giving me a glance. But she always did as she was asked, and would sit where she was put, eat what was laid in front of her, and toilet when she was told.

Around the time of the Lockerbie bombing in 1988, I was asked if I wanted to cover some evening shifts at the home where Enid and some of the other patients on my pickup round lived, by Carol, the home's owner. Outpatient ambulance work was not well paid, and as I only worked during the day, I accepted. The job just involved basic care for the 10 or so residents, making their sandwiches for tea, then bathing the men and putting them to bed before finishing at about 9pm. Only a couple of my brood here were also collected by me during the day, but as time went on I learnt more about them, often from Carol and the other staff, but of particular interest to me was Enid's story. What I learnt horrified me, branding itself into my mind to never forget.

Enid Emily Preston was born in Aston, Birmingham, on 22 June 1898, 3rd child of George and Emily Preston, wealthy owners of Prestons men's outfitting shops based around the Birmingham district. Shortly after entering the world, the family moved to Handsworth and took residence in a large 7 bedroomed victorian house complete with maid. George, her father, was a strict presbyterian who ruled the roost with an iron fist of which Enid and the five other children were reputed to have been in fear of. There had been a seventh child but he died at a young age, being of a sickly disposition. Strictly religious, they would be found at church every Sunday, dressed in their best outfits, bonnets and shoes.

Enid enjoyed the trappings of a monied upbringing; fine

clothes, holidays every year at the sea, steam train travel, and good food. And she was educated, attending schooling in Birmingham until she was 15, much later than the ordinary folk. She was a happy girl too, spending her time with her 3 younger sisters and 2 elder brothers often to be found playing in the warm English summer countryside as was then, or building snowmen in the cold winter times, oblivious to the hardships that the average folk of Birmingham endured; industrial smog, little money, no heating, poor sanitation, few clothes, and a plethora of poverty induced disease. She was particularly close to Wilfred, her brother who was less than a year older. The two of them were reported to be inseparable, and where one was found so too would be the other.

Enid matured into a very attractive young lady, with long blond hair and a slim figure. It was said that she never once needed to wear a corset, as her natural figure made her look as if she was. She cared for the younger siblings, often helping her mother in the kitchen, and performing the chores her father set. And as she grew into her teens, her fathers sharp tongue towards her mellowed, although she would still witness his hand strike them regularly, and her on rare occasions, not for her actions, but for his own self gratification.

Here the story becomes unclear, suffice to say, that at the tender age of 16, around the outbreak of The Great War, Enid became pregnant. There had allegedly been no boyfriend; no one who would put their hand up and admit to becoming the father. But someone knew the truth, and rumours abounded; one said she was raped by her father, who'd been making sexual advances towards her for some time and she'd always managed to evade them before. The other that she was raped by a local known man of poor character who preyed on Enid as she walked home alone, unusually, from a friend's house. Yet another said that her relationship with Wilfred became just too close, and that they'd started a sexual affair, under the cover of a simple sibling closeness. But from whatever cause, Enid was pregnant, in an Edwardian era, with a strict Presbyterian Victorian father, who could not and would not take the shame and depravity, that *she* had brought upon the family. And so her life was to change forever.

Two weeks after the outbreak of World War 1, on 12th August 1914, as far as anyone was concerned, Enid disappeared. Her father told her brothers and sisters that Enid had taken up a place as companion to a wealthy wife and family in the north of England, and that she wouldn't be back. Allegedly the posting had come up at short notice, was ideal for her, if she left without delay, and so caught a train from Birmingham that same evening. Clearly Enid's siblings would have thought this strange that she hadn't mentioned it before, but no one would question their father. Wilfred was especially mystified by the lack of information surrounding the closest person on his earth vanishing. So they took it as said. Her mother remained quiet, throughout the whole ordeal, apparently to be seen dabbing the corners of her eyes when the subject came up and turning her face away from the children.

Of course, there was no wealthy northern family in need of a companion, no posting, and no train journey. The shame of a daughter, pregnant and out of wedlock brought upon George Preston, or so he felt, took him to committing Enid into the local workhouse. Erdington House, formally, prior to 1912, The Aston Union Workhouse (and later Highcroft Psychiatric Hospital) was where she would spend the next 74 years of her life. Even now, as I write this, I find the injustice very emotive.

From the outset, she lost her pretty clothes, the delicious foods, the travel, her comfort and all those trappings she'd had. Her hair was cut short, she was clothed in the same filthy outfits the others 'inmates' had. Others being paupers, idiots, tramps, seniles, lunatics and imbeciles, as mentioned before. Her only 'crime'? Becoming pregnant out of wedlock and in a society where rape either didn't exist or was the 'fault' of the female. And so Enid's institutionalisation started. Being classed as the other inmates, her talents and skills were ignored. She was not allowed to do anything; no mental or communication stimulation, no visits (after all, potentially only her father knew she was there), no means of personal progression. At the time I new Enid, at the age of 90, she had been transferred to the community accommodation I picked her up from some 3 or 4 years before, but by now was not capable of using a knife and fork, or dressing herself. she couldn't tie her shoe laces, couldn't read or write and couldn't feed herself.

In 1984, at the age of 86, purely by chance, Enid's great niece, 35 year old Caroline Owens, came upon the name Enid Emily Preston by chance when she worked for the local health services. Her mother had spoken of Enid fondly to her as a child and the name struck a cord. Over the next few weeks she probed further and discovered a labyrinth of deceit and lies that had led to the poor woman losing her dignity, her future, her very life, and being committed 'for life', for something she likely had no control over. By this time, Wilfred and Enid's other brother, Albert were dead, having been killed in The Great War, and only Winifred and Agnes still remained, as the youngest sister Mary, had passed some years earlier of cancer. Caroline's investigations revealed that it was recorded that Enid delivered a baby girl in March 1915. That was as far as the records went. No one knew what happened to the baby, or even if she was still alive. It is, however, likely that this little girl was taken off her young mother straight away - another punishment from an Edwardian system that had no compassion for her plight. I cannot even begin to think of the suffering and immeasurable hurt this must have given this frightened, innocent child. Further rumour also emerged that George Preston was a patron of the Workhouse, supporting and funding its work, no doubt using it as advertising for his business. But now, in 1988, time had taken its toll, and things were more than too late. Enid was now so institutionalised that she would never integrate back into society.

Following this discovery in the 80's, she started having visits from her rediscovered family. They showed her photographs, and talked to her about her past. They spent part of every day with her for months. But it was no good. As before, she neither spoke to them, nor acknowledged their very existence. She didn't recognise her own sisters, and didn't respond to the memories and stories they shared with her in a bid to get some kind of a reaction. Even the mention of Wilfred produced nothing. Enid, had been systematically brainwashed. Her body language and facial expression, remained as they always had; blank and unremarkable. No communication, no smiling. Everything had been taken away from her, and she had not the tools anymore to enjoy any part of life.

Winifred and Agnes had remained very close, particularly as they were the only remaining siblings. Their visits went on for some time in the hope that one day Enid might recognise or at least say something. But they grew weary at her lack of response, and following the death of Winifred, Agnes, now elderly and frail herself, with poor eyesight and mobility, gave up on trying anymore and once again, Enid was abandoned and left alone. Late the following year, in 1989, Enid Emily Preston died subsequent to a fall at the home she lived in, then developing pneumonia in hospital from which she did not recover. She was 91 years old. She died alone. There was no one with her when she passed, and her funeral was also sparsely attended; the home owner, Carol and her son, and a couple of staff from Highcroft, all wearing the traditional black. And so they should have been, for this wasn't a happy occasion. It wasn't a celebration of her life. It was the mourning of the theft of one. She was cremated at Witton Cemetery, Birmingham, with no interment or scattering of her ashes, no head stone and no mark that she ever existed, and no one will bring her flowers to remember her by. At her funeral however, there was a particular bouquet . On it, the inscription read,

"Dearest Aunt Enid. For the pain you endured, and the life that was taken away from you, may the angels show you a much better place than you were shown by your fellow men. God bless."

CHAPTER 7. DEATH IN THE TOWER BLOCK.

When I got transferred to Sutton Coldfield Ambulance station in 1988, the opportunity heralded a place full of excitement. It was long known for producing quality emergency work without the time wasting callers that plagued Henrietta Street. Oh sure, I'd had a good start at 'The Street' and already liked the place, but now I'd got a move to Sutton, I was pleased at how much friendlier the place was to newbies. Besides, it was within walking distance to where I lived, which was really handy as I hadn't a car at the time. I could even come home for lunch during my split shift 2 hour break.

Sutton Station was a relatively small building, having been built, I'm guessing, around the sixties or seventies. Single story with the mess room at one end of a long corridor and the two offices at the other, one for the gaffer, Ray Cooper, and the other for the admin girl. Everywhere was Parkay flooring and flock wallpaper, but the place had a nice feel about it and was always friendly. The garage had room for about three ambulances and the night shifts cars, all of which were cleaned almost every shift. I remember one of the blokes, Tony, saying to me once that there was no excuse for any ambulanceman to have a dirty car. Another advantage the station had was a pit in the one corner, as the mechanics did some repairs there at a time before I started. With the state of the cars I was to subsequently drive for the next few years, this pit would prove to be invaluable. In fact the eighties rebuilt or cleaned most guys cars in one shape or form. Chelmsley Wood ambulance station, located some 15 to 20 miles away was where the mechanics and all their gear were based. It was reputed that on nights when things were quiet, no end of resprays and engine rebuilds went on.

The guys that worked the Sutton patch on the emergency ambulances were a jolly flock, and the place was alive with laughter, banter and constant jokes played upon each other. Here were another bunch of true characters that will never be replicated. Fred 'Freddie' Winterfield, Guy 'Sticky' Stickland, Stuee Mullet, Tony Allice and Stevie Bantock to name but a few, who between them produced more laughs than you could shake a stick at and cast the environment into an irreplaceable one. Often the jokes were at the expense of one of the lads, but everyone gave as good as they got. No one became offended, and antics were gotten away with that would now surely be imprisonable, let alone sackable.

From early on in my outpatient career, I knew that my destiny lay in the front line; doing the emergency calls and being at the forefront of the blood guts and gore. As I mentioned earlier, outpatient work bored me, and being young and inexperienced, I didn't value the foundation that it was forming for me. I sought the high life, as I saw it. And one way of getting a taster, was to ride 'third man' with the front line crews. This involved initially asking the front line staff if I could go out with them, usually on my days off, sometimes after shift finish, and occasionally during my 2 hour lunch break. And in the days virtually before health and safety, this saw me sitting on one of the two stretchers of, usually a 3 litre V6 sliding door Ford Transit, complete with rotating blue beacons atop, and two tone air horns. In the summer, the sliding doors were open at speed, usually with either the driver or the attendant shouting to the frightened motorists.

"Get out the fuckin' way", and "You blind, love?" And the more popular, "what? Ain't we big enough for you mate?"

This was the era where they got away with this sort of behaviour. No complaints ever came in, as the public motorists saw themselves as the stupid drivers they obviously were.

All the guys, and I say guys, because they were all blokes apart from one woman, had two speeds; stationary and flat out, and with the invent of the 3 litre engine, over its predecessor, the old 2 litre, these were quick bits of kit. Proper ambulances that produced more excitement for me than a cage full of nubile virgins. It was, simply put, bloody fantastic! It seemed that every job saw severed limbs, or severe entrapments, with cardiac arrests every week and the occasional multiple stabbing with the hand grenade thrown in (pardoning the pun).

One man that springs to mind more than most for his driving was Ron 'Turbo' Smythe. Turbo wasn't nicknamed Turbo for no reason. A tall man originally from Staffordshire, and with the accent to accompany, he was slim with a 'Hulk Hogan' type moustache. Ron had a great sense of humour and often worked with Sticky. I loved working with these guys, and still consider that today it was an immense privilege. I learned so much of the basic principles from them that are as apparent today as they were then; simple common sense stuff.

On one occasion, as third man, Raven 3, our call sign, was haring up Boldmere Road, Sutton, on an emergency 999 call, at over 60 mph, twice the speed limit, when we came upon vehicles slowing for a set of red traffic lights. I was always perched on the stretcher in the rear saloon with my arms resting on my knees into the centre and looking through to the front. I expected Ron to ease off. I was wrong. He continued, mounting the pavement.......on the wrong side of the road to avoid the oncoming traffic, negotiated them almost, dare I say it, skilfully, then dropped back to our side of the road in the middle of the red traffic lights, two tone horns still blaring. Sticky slid the sliding door open and shouted at the poor motorists.

"Get out the way! Can't you idiots see its Turbo behind the wheel?"

And even though the wearing of seat belts became law in 1984 in the UK, no one wore them in these ambulances four years later.

We were en route to the report of someone unwell in Castle Vale, a northern suburb of Birmingham, and one of the less desirable areas to have to go to. I'd been an insurance agent in this area before joining the ambulance service, and I actually found most of the residents of this huge estate to be lovely. But in the ambulance service we often see the issues that most do not; drugs, alcohol, assault, rape and any number of other human initiated problems. However, our current call, was to an elderly female who had dialled 999, giving little and confusing information over the phone. It was a stinking hot day in June, and I guess the temperatures would have been up in the high 20's. Turbo negotiated our way through the labyrinth of driveways and blind cul de sacs until we reached Beech Tower. Now even by Castle Vale's standards, Beech Tower was abysmal. A 20 odd storey council tower block built in the 1960's to 'successfully' house 80 families. They started out well, in an era where people were proud and shared the cleaning of the communal hallways, and planted flowers outside, chatting to each other and helping with baby sitting etc. But times had changed. Fewer people cared about their neighbours anymore; out had moved many of the good people years before, and in had moved drugs, prostitution, barking Rottweilers on the balconies, dumped mattresses in the foyer and bags of rotting rubbish littered the hallways because many people just couldn't be bothered anymore. They had become the failure they were destined to be. The trouble is, there's another saying in the ambulance service. 'You can take the scum out of the gutter, but you can't take the gutter out of the scum.'

When they knocked these tower blocks down some years later around the turn of the 21st century, private housing built hundreds of ultra modern apartments in their place, multi coloured and very nice. I know, because following a marriage separation I moved into one. Only to live near a man of my age who'd spent most of his adult life in prison, and was destined to go back there, dealing drugs from the very handout that was designed to get him back on his feet. I rest my case. But you get the image, I'm sure.

So, we arrived at the tower block. The patient lived at number 89, and after negotiating the black bin bags in the foyer, Sticky pressed the lift button with his pen as was customary. Here was another little tip I learned in the tower blocks. Locals smear spit, faeces, sperm, urine and blood across the buttons because apparently it's funny. So you don't press any buttons with your finger. Oh, and you don't suck the end of your pen either. After the statutory couple of minutes wait for the lift, hearing it scraping its way down the shaft, there was a moments pause before the door very slowly opened. Out walked an elderly couple, in a very nonchalant and natural way, despite there being an unwrapped soaked and faeces smeared fresh nappy on the floor, and the smell of urine was over powering. These people had to live in these conditions all day, every day. They were the proverbial inner city slums, made so by a small percentage of people who produced these appalling conditions for the other good folk who resided there. The lifts never gave the floor of the flat you were looking for, only the floor number, so Turbo asked the old couple as they were walking past us which floor 89 was on. Their answer headed us up to the top floor, and after the lift trundled its way up the shaft having given me that, 'Is this gonna get us there or would I have been better walking up the stairs?' moment. But we successfully got out on the top floor and walked towards the door we were looking for. Sticky remembered he'd been here before.

"Bang hard for the hard of hearing, then you can be sure that if they don't answer, they're dead or out." Yep, made sense. Sticky attacked the door, followed by Turbo looking at him with mouth agape.

"Fookin 'ell Sticky. You used to be a rent man or what?"

"Nah", said Sticky, "I bin 'ere before. She's a deaf old bat".

To which he hammered on the door again. From deep in the flat came a reply.

"Ok love, I'm coming."

Following which she started a conversation with us even though we couldn't hear a word she was saying. Turbo started laughing.

"Shut the fuck up, Turbo", Sticky got out quickly, "or you'll start me off".

Turbo and Sticky were renowned for starting each other laughing at the slightest thing. The hallway subdued into a silence as we heard the shuffle of dragging footsteps approach the door. She unlocked it top, middle and bottom, then opened it revealing an elderly lady bent over with arthritis, and having hearing aids in both ears. She had a bright smiling face and took one look at Sticky exclaiming that she remembered him from a previous visit. I looked through into the hallway and saw it was cluttered with boxes, piles of newspapers tied together with string, an old bird cage, piles of dining room chairs stacked on top of each other, and any other number of clutter. I was hit by a musty, stale smell of unclean house, and unwashed person. We all followed her slowly down the hallway and into the lounge, where I immediately noted the view of surrounding Birmingham from being this high up. It was obvious she wasn't on deaths door, so as the other two briefly looked around the room, I thought I'd open the conversation.

"What a lovely, view".

This fell on deaf ears and she didn't reply. Sticky, now shouting, carried on.

"WHAT'S THE MATTER LOVE? WHY'VE YOU CALLED FOR AN AMBULANCE". She turned to him,

"Umm?" she said,

"I suppose you want to know why I've called you, don't you?"

Turbo piped up, in a soft hushed tone.

"No love, not really, we love coming 'ere on a Saturday afternoon. I must remember to bring the missus".

Sticky looked at him with a smile starting, at which point, still following the lady, in the clutter of her flat he tripped over an old fashioned horse hair foot stool, the square, very heavy type rarely seen these days. It had seen better days with the stitching having gone in one corner and the horse hair bulging out. He grabbed the arm of the settee and managed to keep his footing, but was spotted by the lady.

"I'm sorry about that love," she started, "I've been meaning to throw it out for ages."

She turned back round and walked towards the kitchen.

"Well here," lunged Turbo, "Let me help you." As she turned away, he picked up the weighty stool, nearly breaking his back, and threw it out of the open window. 20 floors up.

Sticky's mouth was agape for a second, before he burst out

laughing, quickly stifling it as the old lady turned round, but didn't see what had happened. My thoughts quickly turned to who the missile might have killed below. I moved rapidly to the window, where my actions were echoed by Sticky, who by now was giggling like a child.

"Turbo, you fuckin' twat. You've done it now. You might have killed some fucker."

"No it's all good", I returned, with somewhat of a sigh of relief, having looked out the window and seen the stool in the middle of the road below, splattered and exploded, but fortunately not on top of any one or any car.

The lady, Iris, turned round clearly aware something had happened but didn't know what, and after eyeing us slightly suspiciously for a second, continued.

"It's Cyril. I think he's dead".

"Bloody 'ell" said Turbo in a hushed tone. "You mean we've been here larking around and all the time 'er old mans croaked it in the bedroom. Oh shit". Sticky went into compassionate mode. He put his arm around Iris's shoulder, who sniffed.

"What makes you think he's passed Iris, and where is he?" He said. She started crying and reached for her hanky, conveniently located as all elderly ladies did then, up the sleeve of her thin blue cardigan. After blowing her nose lightly, she continued.

"He's in the bedroom. I didn't think he looked himself yesterday, and I went to wake him this morning but I couldn't. He wouldn't talk to me and he's not moving. He's never done that before".

We all feared the worst, but before she'd finished telling Sticky the story, Turbo had already gone into the bedroom. He reappeared seconds later, and with me and Sticky facing, but with Iris having her back to him, he took his fore finger and drew it across his throat, meaning Cyril was dead. Death in the ambulance service was managed at this time by getting the doctor to come out to certify or pronounce death on the body and the police were required because until otherwise proven, the scene was one of a crime, although in most cases of course, death was of natural causes. Sticky sat Iris down and suggested he put the kettle on, to which she nodded approval. He started to say how sorry he was for her loss, and I became aware that Turbo, unbeknown to Sticky, was smiling and trying to subdue a laugh.

Sticky started to say that the doctor would have to be called, but didn't get it out before he was abruptly interrupted by Turbo.

"Don't worry love, we'll sort Cyril out for you. We'll take him with us and make sure he gets sorted."

Sticky's face told a picture. He obviously thought Turbo had lost the plot. And so did I. Laughing at this poor woman's grief, then stealing the body? He disappeared back into the bedroom, and after Sticky had put the kettle on, reappeared behind Iris holding up a dead budgie. It all fell into place with Sticky and myself. I turned my head to hide my smile, but ever the professional, Sticky kept it going.

"Iris, have you thought about funeral arrangements?"

I was beginning to lose it, and then as now, when I start laughing, I can't stop.

"Hmmmm. I didn't know you could have budgerigars buried. Do I just contact the Co-op like I did when my Frank died." She said.

I knew it was coming, when, sullen faced, Sticky continued,

"Was Frank your cat?" Turbo left the room.

"Ooo no", she continued, "he was my little Yorkshire Terrier. I phoned the ambulance when he died last year, and you boys told me to ring the undertakers. Strange though, they said they wouldn't come out."

CHAPTER 8.
THE RACE.

The summer of 1989 was a hot one; full of long, warm evenings, with warm fragrancies filling the air, and butterflies and bees happily going about their business. I loved these days and used to really look forward to working third man with the lads from Sutton on a Friday evening after work from 6 o'clock. It was always a fabulous atmosphere and the banter was just great. We'd often end the evening shift by a visit to the chippy, and the jobs were always quality. I was virtually guaranteed of a stabbing or a serious road accident. These were the days before air bags and safe cars, where speeds were higher by the mere fact that traffic numbers were fewer, so car verses tree often resulted in entrapment, and the associated blood, guts and gore that I found so exciting. This was an era where ambulances were really needed by the callers, not just because someone had cut themselves shaving. Unbelievable, I know, but yes, a real call to a man who cut himself shaving following a hot bath, and was 'treated' using an ice lolly from the freezer applied to the wound. Or the lady who wanted the channel changing on the television, and couldn't figure the remote out.

One extraordinary Friday evening involved a multiply stabbed and murdered woman on a pavement, and the rampaging murderer brandishing a hand grenade and holding up a bus. Like I say, all in a typical Friday evenings work at Sutton Coldfield in the late 80's.

As has already been eluded to, the banter that went on amazes me even today. Much of it was between Phil and his mate Stan. Stan was stationed at Henrietta Street, and the two had a long history of friendship through the job. I think at one time they were crew mates who had then become key figures in the union. But they also had this 'one-up man-ship' thing going, which became relentless. Their shifts coincided and often if one was at one hospital handing over a patient, the other would roll in. Favoured jokes played on each other included removal of all equipment from the back of the other's vehicle whilst they were inside the hospital, piling it up on the driveway in front of the bonnet. Another one done was to turn all the lights and siren switches on, which did nothing until the unaware crew returned to the vehicle and switched on the ignition, when all hell broke loose with the noise so loud in the confines of the casualty entrance, that it would bring the staff outside to see what 'the emergency' was. And there was never any worry or fear of getting into trouble for some of the antics either, partly due to the two of them being feared union reps, and partly because playing jokes and larking around was the done thing in this era, and the gaffer, Ray, always turned a blind eye.

One of those warm, sunny Friday evenings I was riding third man with Phil and Freddie. Sutton had recently taken delivery of a new 3 litre V6, 5 speed Ford Transit, which then was seen as the mutt's nuts of ambulances. This thing was comfortable, quick and handled well, and everyone wanted to work in it. It replaced the older mark 2 sliding door Fords. We'd eaten some tea around 7 o'clock on the station, and whilst I sat down to watch the television with Freddie, Tony drove his car into the station garage to wash it, as was customary. The emergency phone rang and Freddie answered it, spoke briefly to Metro Control, then replaced the receiver and walked towards the door into the garage, grabbing my attention as he brushed past me.

"We got a fitter on Holland Road. You comin?"

I grabbed my florescent jacket, and walked after him.

"Yeah thanks Fred, whereabouts on Holland Road?

Fred was a tall slim man aged, I reckoned, about 50. He was quite camp in his mannerisms; his walk and the way he held a cigarette. He had a great sense of humour and I found him very funny. I liked him. We all liked him. He was always laughing and joking and never once did I ever see him angry or curt. I used to wonder how he ever remained sensible at the times it was needed. In fact I don't think he could be. He always made me cringe and smile at the same time when he used to leave his business card, for his antiques emporium he used to run on the side, on the sideboards of the old people we used to go out to, on the basis that, he'd say, 'they'll croak it soon, and when the family clear the house out, they'll give me a call and I'll get some bargains on this lot. Some nice stuff here.'

I jumped into the rear of the Transit and Fred into the passenger seat, as Phil brushed the last of the water off his car with a chamois leather he had in his hand, before joining us in the drivers seat. The engine fired up, and with a cigarette sticking out of the corner of his mouth, we roared off the station, and headed towards the location on Holland road, my heart pounding and my breathing racing with excitement. The patient had recovered by the time we arrived a few minutes later, but it was agreed that we'd pop him to the hospital for a check up anyway.

We pulled in to Good Hope Hospital where there was one ambulance already parked up. We all jumped out and Fred and myself went inside the department to handover the patient. Phil sauntered over to the drivers side of the other ambulance, obviously to chat to them, and a couple of minutes later we joined him. Phil, and Stan, the driver of this other ambulance were deep in friendly heated chat. I could hear Stan's voice first as I neared them both,

"I don't give a shit if it is a Ford, I'm fuckin' tellin' ya, The Beast is quicker", ending his statement with a bit of a laugh. 'The Beast', was the nick name given to the vehicle him and his crew mate were in. I remember it well; a 1987, D reg 3.5 litre V8 Freight Rover. They were pretty quick in a straight line, but had the cornering capability of a soggy wet sponge, making them fast, but with 'interesting' handling. On the motorway, it was indeed, good for 110 miles an hour, but then, so was the new Ford. Phil continued the conversation.

"Nah mate. Look, 'ave you ever driven one of the new Trannys?" The question was quick and rhetorical. "No you ain't cuz Henry (meaning Henrietta Street ambulance Station) ain't got one 'as it? So ya don't know, and as per fuckin' usual, Stan, yah talking out yar arse"

I knew Stan briefly when I'd spent a little time at Henrietta Street trying to go out with the emergency crews before returning back to Sutton. I'd found him arrogant and unfriendly and steered clear of him generally. As Freddie and myself approached him and Phil, Stan acknowledged Fred, but ignored me, making me feel embarrassed and giving me a sense of not belonging to the group that I so desperately craved. Stan snapped back at Phil.

"Well, my friend, there's only one way to prove which truck is quicker. A race. Put ya money where ya mouth is son and let's do it. 5 quid says we'll beat you fuckers from Holy Trinity Church back to Sutton station.

Without hesitation, Phil agreed, and with haste him and Freddie returned to our Transit with me in tow jumping back into the rear and sitting down. I had a feeling this was going to be a bit of a rough ride so for the first time, I put a lap belt around myself. And with a complete disregard for contacting ambulance control or what jobs may have been lined up for us, both vehicles departed for the start line. We drove up Rectory Road to the T junction at the top and both vehicles pulled out left onto Coleshill Street, opposite the church, which was quiet; good job really when you consider that both vehicles were now side by side pointing down the hill, us on the correct side of the road, and Stan on the wrong side!

With the front windows down, Freddie reached forward and on went the blue lights with the sirens breaking the relative quiet followed by Phil shouting 'three......two.....one......GO!' And with a roar of the engines, both vehicle hurtled off down the hill side by side. Now anyone who knows this section of road will know that it's a straight road, with a set of traffic lights at the bottom of the hill and cars parked on both sides of the road for its length. Given the same circumstances now, this would not be possible; too much traffic and lots of maturity and common sense. But this was 1989, and the threat of losing a bet was far more important than providing emergency care to the public of the West Midlands.

Speeds increased and the traffic lights loomed ever nearer....and were on red. In the rear of the saloon I was starting to get a little uneasy. I could feel myself tensing and wondering if, this time, these guys were going just too far. Fortunately, no cars were coming towards Stan's ambulance, and nothing lay in front of us, but neither vehicle was slowing for the lights. But as if on cue, the beautiful amber light appeared, and to green they went, as we both sped across the line, still gaining speed. I wondered at that point what the stationary cars at the traffic lights to our left and right would think, seeing two ambulances screaming across the junction, blue lights and sirens blazing, obviously off to save lives at a house burning down, or a vehicle accident with death and destruction hanging out of the car. But of course the truth was much less dramatic.

On and on we went, further and faster, and by now there were cars coming towards Stan who were driving up on the pavement in sheer horror to get out of his way. Stan by now was a full vehicle length ahead and threatening to pull in front of us. Phil shouted out that he wasn't going to let him in because he knew that we'd never be able to overtake them in the mile or so that was left to station. I could see a car rounding the corner in front of us heading in Stan's path that didn't appear to be going up the footpath. I could almost hear the cursing in their cab and was witnessing a stand off in front of my very eyes; car verses ambulance. Who would give in first? The stakes were high and I guessed it wouldn't be Stan. Sure enough at the last second the car mounted the pavement but not before Stan came off the gas enough to lose his vehicle length advantage on us, and through we went to take the leading position. We straightened on to Ebrook Road doing, I'd guessed about 80 miles an hour. I say 'guessed' because there was no way I'd got the guts to take my eyes off the road and on to the speedometer. For here the road narrows due to the parked cars on either side, forcing Stan back to drop in behind us. And from this point on we all knew he was doomed because he'd never be able to get around us. And sure enough we pulled into towards Sutton Ambulance Station the victor. Phil and Fred were whooping with joy and victory, and of course were the first to jump out of the truck and rub it in that Stan and his mate were the losers. They didn't take their loss lightly, blaming it on the parked cars and the conditions. The truth, of course, was that the two vehicles were pretty well matched, but this episode demonstrated what was done in this era. Really, a total disregard for everyone's safety, in the name of larking about for fun. And with this type of driving it was more by luck than judgement that an accident hadn't ensued.

CHAPTER 9. THE MIND PLAYS TRICKS.....

After a year or so at Sutton station, I took a promotion and moved back to Henrietta Street, but still serving the non-emergency community. Working split shifts meant a long day with a break in the middle that was long enough to be boring, but short enough to not be able to do anything constructive, or go anywhere. So the opportunity to move to a better shift pattern with a day off in the week was a move upwards as far as I was concerned, even if it meant a longer commute into the city.

These early days left me with frustration at working on the out patient sector, and the thought of front line provided me with adrenaline fuelled excitement. Being single and still living at home, I was spending a large percentage of my time riding 'third man', and gaining valuable experience of emergency work that I was subsequently moving towards. I just couldn't get enough of it.

A couple of months in from the start, and the jokes with the emergency guys were starting that I hadn't yet, by coincidence, seen and managed a body. The media portrays bodies as looking as if they're alive but just asleep, but I wasn't so sure, and the thought of a deceased person filled me with uncertainty, and left me with a head full of questions; what *would* they look like, and how, as a rookie, would I react at the sight? My questions and intrigue were about to be answered.

It had been a tedious August Friday, that I hadn't looked forward to at all, as it had been my turn to man the ulcer clinic run. We all had to take our turn with this putrid task of taking mundane, unexciting patients with smelly, dripping and dirty dressings in desperate need of change to the hospital. We waited with a cup of coffee, then returned them back, albeit now with a far more pleasant odour, to their armchairs, sticky slippers and walking frames. Gratitude often came in the form of thank-you's and a couple of boiled sweets that had been in their pockets for some time. Most of these patients were diabetic, which had lead to their poor circulation and subsequent ulcers, and the dressings of the time seemed to be little more than absorbent padding and crepe bandages. So after a few days of heat and oozing pus, the smell became disgusting. One lady had legs so bad, that she kept her feet inside plastic bread bags, to prevent her slippers becoming completely sodden with a vile mixture of pus and blood. But her methods failed miserably, leaving the carpet by her easy chair crusty and mushy under foot, and the house with a putrid odour of rotting flesh. Eight ulcer clinic patients in the rear of a passenger ambulance, in the heat of the summer subjected me to an indescribable assault on my senses of hellish proportions that made even the most hardened ambos wretch from time to time. The patients knew it, and harboured all the embarrassment of such, constantly apologising. When working with Jeff Fentley it became a bit of a game with me as the driver to turn the heating up to full in the rear saloon, close the adjoining door, and waiting to see how long it was before he darted back into the front, sticking his head out of the passenger window to vomit. Oh how we laughed........

"I'm sorry dear about the awful smell", Mrs Wright would say each time I stepped over her threshold. "I've tried air freshener, but it doesn't seem to do any good. I'm most awfully embarrassed", she'd go on to say, her eyebrows sagging heavily and the corners of her mouth turning down at the edges, as she stared at the floor with total despondency.

"Oh don't worry Doris", I'd reply with a cheerful tone, "it's not too bad really".

"Oh you are kind dear" she'd go on. But she knew I was just being nice. What she probably didn't see was the few moments I stood at her front door before I pressed the bell, to try to steel myself and acclimatise to what I was about to be faced with.

Despite having taken my turn with the ulcer clinic run, I'd had that excited feeling this Friday; like when you know they herald the start of the weekend where parties and drinking usually abound for young people. But for me the excitement was different. Fridays meant Friday evenings followed by Saturday late shifts of riding 'third man', on the front line where I knew we'd get at least one or two 'juicy' jobs. Was it going to be a stabbing, or a car into a tree? I just hoped it would be something, as I used to get despondent if the weekend finished and we'd had very little to write home about.

Having finished my day shift at Henrietta Street, and with the stench of rotting ulcers still pungent in my nostrils, I washed my ambulance and parked it alongside the other out patient vehicles at the bottom of the garage. I walked past the front line motors with a glint of nervousness in my belly, as I looked at the blue lights that represented what I so wanted. I wasn't sure which shift was on 'lates' that day but hoped that it was C shift, who had been really helpful and friendly, and with whom I'd started to develop a rapport. Walking down the corridor and turning into the mess room, I was greeted with an air of relaxation. It was D shift who were on and they were all in, along with an alternating shift crew of which Stan Smith was one half. He was at the snooker table, facing me and about to take a shot. He paused the stroke remaining completely motionless aside of his eyes which glanced up and caught mine. His face didn't acknowledge me as he returned to his shot, giving the distinctive 'click' of the snooker balls over the quiet TV. My heart sank. I felt intimidated by him, and desperately hoped he wasn't part of the next ambulance out as I hated asking to go with him. He always allowed it but insulted me and made me feel inept and a real newbie. Looking back, I think he gained enjoyment from it.

Ted and Paddy were slumped in front of the television with its low volume. I doubted they were even watching it. Most crews just chilled out and listened to the general banter around the mess room, which historically was either a subject of deep intellect, or a scream of laughter, with various people jumping up and demonstrating how they found a job funny, or replicated a drunk who had given them some verbal abuse. Teddie, or Ted, was a tall slim man of about 40, with a very gentle and soft approach. He had a confident air of experience, where nothing ever seemed to phase him. And more importantly to me, he always greeted me with a cheery smile, spoke and acknowledged me as existing, which was important to me at this stage. Paddy Leggitt was so very different to his crew mate; in his late 50's, and carrying far too much weight, he, like Ted, had years and years of experience. But he was sternly old school and accepted change reluctantly. Paddy's clinical skills were strictly old school and where employment could be gained as an ambulance driver with little more than a driving licence. When little to no patient management was required, and all the situation needed was transport to hospital, Paddy was fine in the back of the ambulance, and Ted preferred to drive anyway, on account that his mate's driving was at best appalling, and at worst downright dangerous. But when they had a really sick patient, Ted would jump in the back and hope that Paddy just took things steady. I liked them. They were characters.

They broke down one day in the ambulance which over heated. A breakdown service was dispatched to pick them up and duly arrived, and although a tow truck, it was actually a flat bed rigid truck with two separate ramps that were manually lifted into place by the driver and the vehicle driven up and onto the back of the bed. With a twin cab the driver brought Ted and Paddy back to the station with the broken down ambulance, still able to be started and driven on and off, to the station. It pulled up outside the garage and all the blokes came out from the mess room to see what the excitement was about. The driver, a young bloke of about 21 put the ramps into place and jumped into the ambulance starting it up to reverse it off. Paddy decided to help and took it upon himself to stand at the back and wave the ambulance towards him as if to guide the driver back.

"Yeah come on" shouted Paddy, "back a bit, back a bit more, yeah come on all good". Then one of the other blokes engaged him in conversation about what had happened to break down. Paddy chatted to him but at the same time was still waving the ambulance back and still intermittently shouting,

"Yeah that's good, keep coming, keep coming".

However, not actually looking at where the wheels of the ambulance were positioned on the down ramps and not realising that they were getting dangerously close to the edge of the ramps. He continued waving backwards while looking and chatting to the other bloke about the breakdown. All of a sudden there was a lurch of the ambulance and it fell off the side of the ramps while still only half way down.

"Fuckin' 'ell" shouted someone and Paddy stopped waving; his arm remaining motionless in the air. The ambulance slid off the ramps and landed at a 45° angle stuck up against a road sign which prevented it from falling completely. Sniggering from the blokes started and Paddy quickly started walking away.

"Fuck all to do with me," he said, before quickly disappearing inside to the mess room and hiding. The young lad climbed out of the drivers seat, scratched his head while looking around for Paddy then phoned his boss, where upon a short time later he arrived and sacked the driver on the spot, who then phoned his brother, who also turned up and a fight started in the street. The blokes meantime who had been getting bored after the ambulance fell off the ramps were now retreating back inside and coming out with chairs and mugs of tea to be more comfortable for 'the show'. But not Paddy, who denied everything, kitted up another vehicle and for once was glad to go out on a job. And the cause of the breakdown after all this? Whoever checked the water at the start of their shift hadn't put the radiator cap back on……..but I digress.

At about 9 o'clock, as some of the blokes were dozing off, the silence was broken with the ring of the emergency phone. My heart raced but I desperately hoped Stan wouldn't pick it up. It rang a couple of times and Stan tutted loudly as his eyes flicked upwards momentarily. He turned towards Ted and with his distinctive accent, shouted sarcastically.

"So you wankers gonna get that or what? We're on break". Ted opened his gritty eyes and Paddy jumped up and walked towards the phone. He picked it up and spoke with a cold tone as if the control centre had some kind of audacity to call and disturb them.

"Yep", his opening word thrust out, not as a question, but a statement. Then there was silence for what seemed like ages. I watched Paddy with trepidation and hung on to his every word as the rest of the crew room dozed in the half light. "Uh huh. Ride O". He casually put the phone down, and proceeded to undo his trousers to tuck his shirt in, his fat belly hanging over his belt. He had an air of calm, and clearly to me this case was going to turn into a routine one of little concern. When his clothes were straight, Paddy was joined by Ted, who stood, stretched, yawned and farted loudly. One of the other guys who I'd assumed was asleep, spoke up without opening his eyes,

"Oi, ya dirty fucker!"

And in his happy, smiling fashion, Ted replied.

"My pleasure", before turning towards the door and asking Paddy what the job was.

"Oh it's a cardiac arrest at the Bowlers Arms pub", said Paddy in such a casual way, before turning for the mess room door clearly in no hurry and with no thought for me. I became excited, having already stood up in anticipation.

"You wanna come?" Ted asked. "But if he's in cardiac arrest now, he'll be dead before we get there, so you won't see much".

It never failed to amaze me in these early days how the experienced blokes looked upon jobs which I'd have given my right arm to attend, with such unimportance, as if I would be bored! The prospect of performing CPR, or even just managing a body, was invaluable to my development at this stage in my career. But they just couldn't see it, presuming I was only there for Gucci road accidents and jobs involving guns. I started my timid reply with the low level of confidence I had then.

"Yeah..urm....if that's ok....." I tailed off as by now Ted was out of the mess room and halfway down the corridor towards the garage, his leather soled shoes, standard issue in those days, clicking on the Parkay floor with a pace of some motivation. I followed him guessing if he'd asked me, then I was good to go. In these early days there was an etiquette when riding third man with the crews. Jack had said to me to always ask the lads, and never assume it's ok to go out with them. Show enthusiasm, clean the truck after the job, and make the tea upon return, and I wouldn't go far wrong. Ted was great on this basis, often asking me before I'd asked him. Paddy on the other hand wasn't really bothered either way, if I came out or not.

I was still trying to get my arm into my florescent jacket, whilst at the same time running to catch up with Ted. As I crossed the garage I opened the back door of 'Eagle 3' and jumped in just in time to feel the engine roar into life as we started moving forward before I'd had a chance to sit down. These were still the days when most of the blokes never wore seat belts. Ted, now with a freshly lit cigarette perched in the corner of his mouth, flicked the blue light switch and the two tone air horns as we raced out of the station turning left and left again onto Summer Lane. I loved this bit. I felt important, empowered and like I'd achieved something. 12 months before, I'd been collecting insurance premiums as a boring salesman. Now I was in a speeding ambulance, going to a life and death situation, with cars moving out of way, and red traffic lights being no hinderance to our progress. We overtook the slowing cars as they pulled over having heard the 'two tones', and gently weaved from left to right, slowing occasionally before speeding up with a throaty roar from the V6. A million thoughts were going through my head, the main of which being that I didn't want to screw up, and make a bad name for myself with the blokes. I felt nervous, and a little queasy at what I'd see. A fear of the unknown would always provoke such a response.

Paddy started off some conversation about his allotment. I was not able to concentrate on his words, but he just went on and on with Ted giving the occasional, 'ah yeah', or 'uh hum'. I got the impression he was just about as bored with the topic as I was. Paddy was famed for both his lack of hygiene and his gardening, two subjects which combined to see him sat on the back steps of the station one summers evening crumbling up horse manure with his bare hands to prepare it for his allotment. Having finished he wiped his hands on his trousers, came into the station and proceeded to eat his sandwiches and make a brew, and in his generosity asking us all in the mess room if we wanted one. It was a cheap round for him for not surprisingly no one took him up on his offer.

I remember wondering how an ambulanceman could chat about something so unconnected with what we were about to see. In fairness, in my naivety at the time, years later I realised that with experience came the ability to be able to chat about something bizarrely unconnected with the perceived horrors of what crews were driving towards. Some use it as a way of 'relaxing', others because they want to disconnect with what they have been told they are facing on the basis that many times, when they arrive on scene, events are so very different from what they've been told, so they need to manage as they find and not make pre judgements.

The Bowler's Arms pub lay on the Walsall Road, in Perry Barr. It was an ordinary boozer and although the ambulance service frequented it from time to time for the odd punch up, it wasn't particularly known as a troublesome establishment. Generally serving an older clientele, it had a 'snug' in the bar, and a lounge area towards the back and was situated on the into city side of a duel carriageway leading us to drive past it to perform a U turn at a set of lights some short way up the road. As we passed the dimly lit pub, all seemed normal; a few cars on the car park, and a couple of men chatting in the doorway. But certainly no sense of panic and having turned at the lights we finally pulled onto the car park in front of the building.

It was so very typical of Birmingham pubs of the late 80's; the outside drab and clearly in need of renovation with its shabby faded sign and peeling paintwork. The few car park lights still working, did a poor job of illuminating the area as the warm summer evening light waned. Ted switched off the blue lights, as the two old men in the doorway looked up, clearly not expecting us. I wondered if this was going to be a hoax call, just as Paddy voiced my thoughts. He jumped out first and approached the entrance to the bar, and as I alighted, I heard one of the blokes at the door ask Paddy who we'd come for, which further confirmed our thoughts of a 'mickey', the slang for a hoax call.

"Dunno", said Paddy, "you any idea who called us?", he said with an air of authority.

"No mate", came the reply. "Go ask Rose at the bar. 'Er with the big tits". They both started laughing, and I could hear them continuing the theme of Rose's large breasts, as Ted and me brushed past them carrying a Pneupac resuscitator and a few other bits ready for jumping up and down on someone's chest. Paddy, of course, carried nothing.

Inside, the heavy acrid smell of stale smoke filled the air, and created a blanket of fog that floated lazily, before wisping upwards having been disturbed by our entry. I looked around. There were three or four groups of people chatting, some with drinks poised in their hands. A couple of men stood alone at the bar, with half empty pints in front of them. Quiet laughter that initially came from over in the corner stopped abruptly as the whole place turned to look at what excitement had just come through the door. They paused for a moment as we neared the bar, then resumed their previous stances, and the chatting picked up again.

It was obvious to us all who Rose was; a hugely buxom woman, with a dress that struggled to cover her cleavage. Somewhat over weight, she was a woman in her fifties, I'd guessed, with greasy lank hair, a round fat face with flushed cheeks and a look that would stop a fight. Paddy approached her, as her gaze drew him in.

"Any one call for an ambulance love?" His tone had changed to one that men develop when they talk to a considered pretty woman. I felt sick to think he found her attractive, but as she spoke I slightly warmed to her. In any case, with the cleavage that adorned her front, Paddy never actually looked her in the eye. She had a soft voice with a Somerset accent and reminded me of the dirty chat lines where the voice sounds ever so sexier than the woman looks.

"Oh yes me darlin', it's Sid in the snug over there." She pointed to the far corner. " 'E's bin there all day, which is nuffin unusual for Sid. Eee comes in every day 'bout 2, 'as five or six pints then goes 'ome bout 7. Bu'rye noticed 'bout 6 tha' eed only 'ad 2 pints since ee came in."

We all turned to look at Sid, who indeed was sat in the corner, with an empty beer glass in front of him, his chin resting on his chest and his arms by his sides. The light was poor and I couldn't see too much detail from this distance. But as I approached, I saw his face was purple, and his tongue was swollen and partly out of his mouth with froth around it. I leaned forward to look at his face. His eyes were half open and had dried out with an eerie expressionless look about them. He was motionless and even I could tell he was dead, and not recently either. Paddy had stayed to talk with the barmaid as me and Ted had approached the patient. I heard him speak to her.

"So how longs ee bin like this then love?"

"Oh a couple hours I spose." Then she became a little more stern, "I only noticed cuz I'd poured 'im another pint an sat it on the bar, and look, there it still is. I 'ope he's gonna pay for it. Is ee alright?"

Paddy walked in our direction. With a hushed tone, Ted spoke to confirm my thoughts.

"Well, Sid's had 'is last pint, poor old bugger".

"What d'ya mean poor old bugger?", replied Paddy. "Gasping ya last in front of tits like Roses, whilst supping a pint! Lucky old bugger more like!"

I tried not to smile, as the pub locals had realised what was going on and had shifted their focus our way. I didn't stop to think at the time as to how I was feeling, but later, on reflection, I realised that my first sight and experience of death hadn't given me any grief up to this point, and Paddy's comment of 'black humour' had actually helped to calm me.

Black humour was, and to a large degree still is, the 'one liner' or the joke passed, at times when Joe Public, were they to hear it, would consider it most inappropriate and unnecessary. But I've come to realise its value when used appropriately for de-escalating stressful circumstances. The secret is to make sure the comments hit only the target audience, and no one else. Imagine the scene of the crew who attended the deceased Florence Parks, who some time earlier had passed peacefully in her sleep upstairs. Florence was a well known 'frequent flyer' with the lads from Henrietta Street, and was famous for her outrageous, cheap and nasty wigs, and a plastering of makeup, troweled on, that she wore each time she attended hospital. The family had been requested to remain in the back kitchen with the door closed to save them the upset of seeing their loved one passed. Wig less and bald headed, Florence was being carried downstairs on the carry chair, when one of the daughters popped her head around from the hall to ask if anyone wanted tea, only to be met by two ambulancemen, carrying a chair with a bald body on it, both wearing wigs so audacious, The Gay Pride would have been proud. And in true style, they simply carried on, explaining they had no where else to put the wigs to carry them as their hands were full. And they were believed. Black humour.

As there were no suspicious circumstances to Sid's death, Paddy had volunteered to go and get the carry chair in order for us to get him out to the ambulance and off to the city mortuary as he was in a public place. These days paramedics are qualified and certified to pronounce, or confirm death. But in the 80's this had to be legally carried out by a doctor, so our journey to the mortuary would be extended by stopping off at The General Hospital in Steelhouse Lane. While waiting for his crew mate, Ted gathered Sid's things which lay on the table in front of him; his wallet, paper, pipe, baccy pouch and trilby hat. Then when Paddy returned we lay a blanket over the chair, and once Sid was lifted across, he was wrapped tightly in it. Ted had put a couple of incontinence sheets on the seat of the chair, which in my inexperience, I'd asked why.

"In a moment, you'll smell something," he started. "The blanket has lots of holes in it. The incontinence sheets don't. And seeing as how you'll be cleaning up at the end of this job, we're doing you a huge favour".

I thanked him, and buckled up the straps before the chair was wheeled out. As we neared the door, the hushed silence slowly broke and the chatter returned, fading as the heavy oak door slowly closed behind us. Carried up the steps by Ted and myself, the body was placed on the stretcher. Paddy was already sat back in the front, reaching into his grotty bag which lay between the seats. As Ted put the last strap over Sid to secure him, I watched as his mate pulled out a sandwich, clearly homemade and the thickness of a door stop, rested it on his trousered thigh before reaching back into the bag and pulling out a pot of salt which he proceeded to sprinkle liberally on the inside of what he was about to eat. Paddy had just been handling a body, with every conceivable body fluid oozing out, in the days before barrier gloves and when he'd not washed his hands either. Even Ted, well used to Paddy's habits spoke up.

"Bloody 'ell Paddy!", to which a bitten sandwich was thrust rearwards in our direction with an offer of a bite. Needless to say, we declined.

With far less haste than our outward journey, Ted pointed the ambulance in the direction of the General Hospital, and having given Metro control an update message over the radio, proceeded to get the body inspected by a doctor. I of course sat in the rear saloon on one side while Sid lay on the other, wrapped now loosely in a blanket with just his face showing. I spent the short journey, facing towards the front, joining in with the worthless chat that ensued, continuing Paddy's conversation about his compost heap. But at least now, with my adrenaline spent, I could concentrate a little better than earlier.

By now, well dark, we pulled up outside the casualty entrance, where I assumed the process of pronouncing death would be momentary, and so it surprised me when both of them stepped out. At this I got up and, opening the rear door, jumped out, only to be met by Paddy.

"Not you lad, you need to stay here with the body for continuity purposes. So no one doesn't mess with the body. Me an' Ted will go find a doc. We'll be back in a minute."

The process of managing a body in those days was to get death pronounced on the deceased by a doctor at the hospital, and when they were happy that the poor unfortunate had indeed passed away, the ambulance crew would then drive the short two hundred yards to the city's central mortuary, where during the day, there was an attendant on duty in the premises. But at night time they were on call and usually took well over an hour to come out. So the crews would wait the hour drinking tea and casually chatting to the reception girls at the hospital. Which is exactly what was going on, on this very occasion. Except I didn't know. So Paddy's 'back in a minute', was their prank on the poor subordinate me who was destined to spend over an hour with a body in the back of a dimly lit ambulance with only the lights from outside to illuminate my now eery environment and keep me safe from the ghosts and ghouls that might come and get me.

The first few minutes passed and then boredom crept my way. 'Not a problem', I thought, 'they'll be back in a minute'. So I waited. And waited. And at the point that I thought there was something amiss and that I should go looking for someone, I remembered Paddy telling me I had to stay with the body. But to make matters worse, I now wanted a wee. Why is it that whenever we have the opportunity to use the toilet, we don't want it? But given the circumstances where we can't access the opportunity, we realise we're desperate to go. And the feeling was welling ….

Sat opposite Sid, I looked at his face. It was wrinkled with a days worth of stubble I guessed, and painted a picture of years of hard work in a factory or a foundry. It had seen so much change, and I imagined that although one of 'the lads' in his earlier years, as he'd become older and nearing retirement, he'd been ousted by the younger blokes and cast aside as being useless and no longer an asset to the company, sent to his old age with little more than his pension. His hair was long and unkempt and he'd got an unwashed smell about him. In the poor light, his eye nearest me was half open, and as my imagination started getting the better of me, I wondered if he might open it fully and turn his head towards me like in some 'edge of the seat' horror film. Then again, maybe he'd say something, or suddenly sit up. After all, he hadn't yet been declared officially dead. What if the guys had been wrong and he was still alive? Now I really was starting to get the jitters, and this wasn't helped, when looking closely at his chest I started to convince myself that he was breathing, albeit shallowly, but there was movement. I studied the loose blanket covering his chest intently. Was there movement or not? I decided to get nearer, just to confirm in the bad light that there was definitely no breathing. I leaned forward until I was inches from his chest, when suddenly his bloody arm, held near his chest only by the loose blanket fell off the side of the stretcher and hung down with his hand hovering just above the floor as it swung a couple of times. I shot back away to the safety of my side of the ambulance with a loud cry.

"Ahhhhhgggggg", followed rapidly by me sliding up the stretcher I was sat on to get to the back door. There was no way I was staying in the back with 'Sid, the living dead'. I couldn't get out of the truck quick enough, as I fumbled with the handle, turning it the wrong way first before getting it right and falling out on to the car park as the door flung open, right at the feet of Ted, Paddy, the doctor and casualty sister who all looked at me as if I was on another planet. In my panic, all thoughts of professionalism, and maturity went out the window, as I blurted out that Sid was back from the dead.

"He breathed and tried to strike me with his arm" I continued, rapidly realising by the look of disgust on sister's face that I was making a huge spectacle of myself. Ted poked his head inside the rear of the ambulance as I looked up at him from the ground. He started laughing, when he realised that this was the mind set and overactive imagination of an inexperienced young ambulanceman. Sid was dead, and had been for some time. It was merely the weight of his arm that had set it free from the blanket which had held it in place. The doctor stepped over me climbing in to look at Sid, before I got up, by now feeling really stupid and wishing the hole would open up and whisk me away from this humiliation. Ted's laughter was subsiding, and the doctor, ignoring me, got on with pronouncing death, which in Sid's case was virtually done from five feet away. Sister scowled at me sarcastically, and Paddy remained nonchalant. I think by this time his tiredness and need for the end of his shift had set in and few things were going to be found humorous.

My initiation of the deceased had been a memorable one, and

was to become the first of hundreds more dead people to come. The story floated the mess room for a few weeks and I had to put up with the mickey taking until the blokes bored of it, and someone else's story took over. So with paperwork in hand, I climbed once more into sit opposite my companion for the trip to the mortuary. This time though with the confidence that he was actually dead, as stated by the doctor, and in any-case I had Ted to protect me if he wasn't.

CHAPTER 10. AN AMBULANCE ICON

The rapidly approaching winter of 1989 saw things heat up within the ambulance ranks, the unions and the management. Discord had been growing for some years over the pay disparity between the three emergency services. The Fire Service and the Police had more pay, better conditions, better pensions, and overall a much better deal than we did. Talks started breaking down as the autumn set in, and the unions started threatening industrial action, as the staff were not accepting the offers made of pay increases. I was still working on the outpatient sector and blissfully unaware of the consequences of industrial action. I still lived at home and had little in the way of out goings, but fear set in amongst many of the seasoned blokes who'd seen the strike of '71, where hardship had abounded, and little was gained. And 1989 was long after Maggie Thatcher had seen to it that the British unions would no longer rule the roost. She'd weakened them and taken away their bullying influence, leaving them seemingly little more than a pathetic token gesture. In November, the ambulance services nationally went into dispute, refusing to do anything other than cover emergency calls. We were not on strike on this basis, but wanted to show management that we meant business. The government responded by cutting us off, calling in the military to cover the emergency calls and shutting us out, hoping that without pay, and over the winter time too, we would give in first. And what a winter it was.

Our resolve and morale were very high and the public supported us well. They could see our plight, and gave generously for months into the buckets of those of us that went out onto the streets collecting donations to try and make ends meet financially. For us at Henrietta Street Ambulance Station, local businesses also chipped in with food, supplies and other essentials. A local garage donated a vehicle which we manned around the clock providing our own emergency cover for the people of Birmingham with the help of the local council who provided an office, a phone and the advertising of a number that folk in need of an ambulance crew could phone. It was marginally successful, until the council were told to withdraw the facilities. They were of course, condoning our plight, and with the strength of the management and government against us, we never had a chance from the outset.

I reported to station daily, and teamed up with a couple of blokes to go and stand in a particular spot in the city centre to rattle the tins and shake the buckets. As the days went on, the clothing got thicker, and the temperature got colder. We'd walk to the ramp that lined the entrance to The Bullring Shopping Centre, and there we would stand for the next six hours until fingers, toes and noses had lost all sense of feeling and spirits were drained. But we did have the occasional lifting moment. Two or three times during the day, someone from the station would come round with hot sausage sandwiches and coffee to warm us up and lift our sagging spirits, and at the end of the day, upon return to the station, all the buckets would be emptied onto the big tables and the money would be counted, never failing to amaze how much money we were taking in. It had been decided early on that everyone would get an equal share, regardless of how much money we normally earned. I ended up taking home about my normal wage, but some of the guys with big mortgages just couldn't manage on this, and some left the job, rather than go back to work and turn their backs on their mates.

My 'collecting' buddy was Floyd 'Floydy' Peterson, a military veteran and long standing ambulanceman, and we got on famously. I already knew him well as he and his mate Kelvin 'Kel' Derby, part of C shift, took me out with them, and each time, I had a ball. I looked forward enormously to them being on lates on Fridays and Saturdays just so I could work with them. Floydy was old school. When he'd started as an ambulanceman sometime in 1960's, all he'd needed to get out on the road was a driving licence and a first aid certificate. He had very little in the way modern science understands about qualifications. And yet he had a myriad of both experience and understanding; common sense and intuition which all came together as far as I was concerned to make for someone to whom I aspired. I envied his ability to fathom a patient out, and diagnose with incredible accuracy. He was, who I wanted to become, and taught me as much as any textbook since. Formal education is a modern necessity for sure, but raw experience makes for ability, and that has to be earned over time.

About 65 years of age, and nearing retirement, Floydy was incredibly young at heart and a real womaniser. At five feet six inches, he was usually to be found on the station, either playing scrabble or glued to the slot machine which he seemed to feed as if it was his last day on earth. He'd gloat when the £50 jackpot rattled in his pocket, only to be reminded by Kel that he'd put five times that amount in to win it. He'd reply with a chuntered response through pursed lips which gripped the cigar that usually adorned his mouth.

Floydy had a colourful background and loved to recount stories of his times in the jungles of Borneo where he was the only 'doctor man' for miles, and had to deal with any number of things from amputations to cases of gonorrhoea, demon possessed locals to child birth. I loved to listen almost as much as he liked to tell, cringing at some of his stories such as when, as a young soldier at a native dance, the way to determine whether a girl was clean enough to consider having sex with later in the night, was that after several drinks and dances, he would perform the 'Pantie Shuffle'. This involved, whilst smooching on the dance floor, sliding his hand up and inserting a finger inside her knickers, enough to gather 'scent', then bringing said finger of hand around the back of her head as he hugged her to be in a position to sniff his finger. This I was reliably informed, kept him free of venereal disease for his entire military career. Allegedly. I found him fascinating and he regularly reminded me that he'd delivered over 300 babies. Kel always asked him how many of them had been his, to which Floydy would chunter again under a half breath, reminding Kel to respect him for being an old soldier, and that he didn't understand because he'd never worked in the jungles alone....But it was true, Floydy was flirty with the women, which sometimes caught him out.

Floydy and Kel were called to a report of a distressed woman, who was allegedly locked in a flat unable to get out. When they arrived at the flat in Edgbaston, Floydy being the attendant, knocked on the front door with the cursory raised tone of 'ambulance, hello, anyone about'. The sound of footsteps could be heard along with a female crying. The footsteps got louder, then from the other side of the front door she spoke.

"I can't get out. He's locked me in. There's a bolt on the top of the door. Can you unlock it?" They looked up in unison, and there, sure enough, was a large bolt, locked across keeping her from coming out. The boys were appalled and looked at each other in disbelief.

"Alright love, don't worry", Floydy stated trying to remain calm. He undid the bolt and tried the handle. The door opened and he stepped in through the opening straight in to the lounge. The woman was by now sat on the sofa in the middle of the room sobbing and he walked over, sitting alongside her. She was a young, plain looking woman of about 30, with long hair fashioned into a ponytail. Kel remained in the doorway and surveyed the room, as is often the case with the driver, who has enough detachment from the patient to spot things around the room, and generally be the watchful eye. Floydy put his arm around her shoulder to offer some comfort, and her cries started to subside.

"Now now love, come on, whats all this about hmmm? Come on tell me all about it. Whats your name?" His tone was actually incredibly condescending and in the style of the bloke chatting up a woman in a bar. Kel cringed and waited for the harsh reply, or the slap round the face. But incredibly she nestled in close to him, inclined her head into his shoulder and put her hand on his knee.

"It's Denise. You're such a comfort", she said, "I feel much better all ready". Floydy turned to look at Kel who was leaning on the frame of the front door with his arms folded watching the proceedings and wondering what had occurred. The old boy winked with a wry smile and a raise of the eyebrows to Kel who looked around the room and pondered the cause of the lady's distress. She continued.

"It's my boyfriend you see. He's such a bully and hits me all the time. He locks me in the flat when he goes out and doesn't let me out.

"Ah I see", said Floydy. "Well you don't need to worry now, cuz we're here to protect you". He put his other hand on the side of her face, and she replied by putting her arms around him and squeezing him tight. Kel thought this a little strange and as he looked further around the room noticed 2 vibrators on the table, a large pink one about 10 inches long resembling the shape of a real, albeit large, penis, and a smaller black one which looked like a series of balls stuck one on top of the other, both alongside a pornographic magazine. Kel craned his head to read the name of it and see the pictures, and oblivious to his mate, he read the title 'Big Boy', along with an article entitlement of 'Cynthia likes it big from her fella', and the picture underneath of a naked woman with large breasts bending forwards and being taken from behind by a guy, the picture having a large black star positioned over the erotic bits for top shelf viewing. Kel started to hope that the pictures inside wouldn't have the same censoring, when he became aware that the woman appeared to be getting closer to Floydy, who looked at Kel with the same wry smile as before.

"You'd better go and ask for the Police", Floydy stated, beckoning with his head to Kel in the direction of the exit.

"Ride O", Kel replied, turning and walking back out to the ambulance to use the radio.

As Kel walked away, the woman released her grip on Floydy, stood up and went to the front door where she closed it stating she didn't want the neighbours to hear all her problems. Floydy continued his reassuring patter about how much of a shame it was that a bright, good looking girl as her should be treated so badly, and he'd clearly taken his eye off the ball, succumbing to the woman's ulterior motives as unbeknown to him she'd locked the door from the inside and returned to the sofa where this time she knelt between his legs and attempted to undo his belt. Reality stepped in and Floydy stood up with his arms on her shoulders holding her back. He fumbled.

"Now, er, come on now, Denise, don't do tha...." he tailed off as she made another grab at his trousers. Each time she got further he would release one shoulder to try and stop her with one hand, grabbing at his fly zip, at which point, now less restrained, she would make further advances of removing his trousers. He was losing the battle, and started to run round the settee, shouting

"KEL! KEL! HELP ME!" As he ran, she followed pulling his trousers down around his ankles, bowling him over as if she'd rugby tackled him. Down he went in a frenzy, desperately trying to cover his embarrassment with one hand and fight her off with the other. Denise grabbed his slip-on shoe and off that came, as Floydy managed to get to his feet and off the comedy chase started again round and round the sofa.

"Come on, you know you want it," Denise fired, through angry, gritted teeth. "Fuck me……Come on, screw my brains out and give it to me hard. I want you…" She was like a demon possessed, with a look on her face that scared Floydy to death. Still running, he continued to bleat, "HELP. KELVIN, WHERE THE BLOODY HELL ARE YOU? HELP ME!"

Kel, in the meantime, had gone down several flights of stairs, to sit in the truck and wait for a space on the radio to get his request in for the police to attend as a matter of non urgency. He lit up a cigarette, took a couple of drags, and meandered back into the block expecting to see his crew mate drinking a cup of tea with the placated Denise swooning around him like so many women had done before. But on the second flight of stairs, Kel heard the cries of help, and sprinted upstairs. Of course, coming to the door, and turning the handle at speed, meant his shoulder hit a brick wall and he came to a sudden stop. The noise coming from inside sounded like a scene from The Exorcist, with some demon enriched woman's voice shouting obscenities and requests mingled with male cries for help that could only have come from someone out of breath. Kel bent down and peered through the letter box. The sight made his fear turn to laughter. Floydy was slightly ahead of Denise in the 'round the sofa' race, with a pair of trousers wrapped tightly around his left ankle, no shoes and a pair of spotted underpants that could also have been destined for the southward journey if Denise had made anymore progress. She had also somehow managed to remove her top half clothing during the chase and her breasts were frantically bobbing up and down as her cries could still be heard above Floydy's, who could by now hear the laughter coming from outside of the front door.

"Kelvin, I know you're bloody well outside, and if you don't get yourself in here right now, I'll …..well I'll…..just get the fuck in here."

Kel by this time was in no fit state to kick a door down. He had become hysterical with laughter, the tears rolling down his face, totally unable to speak.

Another 30 seconds passed, by which time Kel managed to compose himself enough to make an attempt to rescue his mate. Still laughing, he stood to his feet, and became aware of someone approaching him from the stairwell. He turned to glance at the figure of a man; a huge man of over 6 feet tall he'd guessed, and no stranger to working out, staring right at him as he got ever nearer. The humour went, and rapidly, as the reality of what was happening dawned on him. This approaching bloke was heading for Kel and the flat. Two and two quickly made four. He was the boyfriend, was a big guy, who appeared no stranger to fighting and violence, and inside the flat was Floydy with no trousers, having a run round the settee with this bloke's girlfriend whose boobs were swinging in the breeze.

'This was going to hurt', Kel thought to himself. Thinking on his feet, he decided to try and talk his way out at least to divert the man away from Floydy.

"Hello mate, you live here do yo……..", before he was interrupted by the giant, who didn't even acknowledge his existence but walked towards the door and just didn't stop as he turned his shoulder slightly as it made contact with the wood. It flung open with some ferocity as the bloke looked around the room. Denise stopped in her tracks.

"Ello babe", she said with embarrassment. Floydy rapidly dragged his trousers back on, grabbed his other shoe and backed away towards the corner anticipating also, that this was going to hurt. Kel had seen his fair share of scuffles over the years, and one thing being part of an ambulance crew taught, is that you stick together no matter what. Kel piled into the room behind the hulk, and braced himself for the one sided punch up that he expected to follow. But completely to everyone's surprise, the guy gently turned to Denise first, took her hand and sat her down.

"Come on bab, you know you're not supposed to do this. These men are ambulance drivers. You know that". Denise started to cry, this time genuinely. He turned to Floydy.

"Mate, I'm really sorry. Denise is sick. She can't help herself. You won't call the police will you?" Kel was flabbergasted, but incredibly relieved that today, he wasn't going home with a broken jaw.

Denise had a severe form of nymphomania for which she was receiving psychiatric help. But her condition was so bad that he'd had to start locking her in for the safety of men outside. The postman, the gas man, the pizza delivery guys; they'd all black listed the flat. So after locking her in, she'd had the idea of phoning 999 to get men 'delivered' so to speak. Floydy played the whole thing down of course, saying that he never once felt threatened, and had the whole thing under control, and that it wasn't as Kel subsequently described it in the mess room. For weeks.

As the dispute rolled on over Christmas 1989 and into the new year, Floydy and I found ourselves standing alongside the same collecting buckets in Birmingham city centre with no light at the end of the tunnel for a return to work. Day after day, we'd stand, as icy blocks, in the biting wind, chanting out our gripes like the miners had done some years before. We got to know some of the regulars who walked past us at the same times every day; office workers scurrying late, police officers walking the beat, and street cleaners pushing brooms. They'd all give us cheery 'hello' and would often drop a few coins into the bucket.

One such chap was a vagrant by sight; long straggly, dirty grey hair which constantly fell over his eyes and had to be pushed aside as he walked so he could see. He had years of beard growth and an odour about him that claimed he'd started growing it around the time of his last bath. A sort of squashed, holed, trilby hat adorned his head, and a heavy brown overcoat sat tightly on his shoulders, tied at the front with some string. Around his neck an expensive looking woollen scarf wrapped tightly into his coat, no doubt given to him by a sympathetic listener. His trousers painted a picture of 1960's free love, being slightly on the short side and a putrid shade of lime green. And on his feet, an odd pair of training shoes, whose soles had almost become detached and flapped as he walked. I say 'walked', but his forward movement was more of a sideways shuffle which matched his hunch to make him look like a slow version of the hunchback of Notre Dame.

Looks, however, can be deceptive, for when he spoke, the most amazing Queen's English would emanate from his lips. His accent was one of a public school upbringing and his intelligence was clearly one of the better universities. He had an incredible gentle, yet intriguing way about him, like he genuinely cared for who he was talking to, and an almost regal aura, that told a story of one who'd come from good stock and fallen on hard times. Every day, at the same time of just gone 10 o'clock, he would approach from the same direction. He'd stop, don his hat, wish us a good day, put a two pence coin in the bucket, and move on. And as the days wore on his chat would increase in volume until we'd talk for ten minutes or so, at which point, he'd say something like, 'good gracious, is that the time? I've held you good people up for long enough, and I've things to do. Cheerio!' and off he'd shuffle into the crowds as if he was sticking to some schedule or other. The reality, as we found out, was quite different.

Tobias Lysander Valentina-Smyth was born into the wealthy Valentina-Smyth family on 13th September 1919 in India. His Victorian father had amassed his fortune on tea plantations and fostered him with a strict religious upbringing. A very bright young man, at the age of 18, he was sent to Oxford University in England to study law, and at the age of 22 he was conscripted into the British army as an officer in an infantry regiment, to fight in World War 2. Following several campaigns, and achieving some formidable bravery medals, he was wounded out of the fighting in 1944, and was sent back to Britain for recovery. After the war, and still contemplating his scars, he started practicing law as a junior, working his way up to eventually see him taking his Bar exams and qualifying as a barrister in 1952. By 1960, his expertise in courtroom prosecution was feared, and he developed a reputation which saw him take on, and win, several prominent cases. But in Toby's words, and to coin a phrase, 'when you get to the top, there's only one way to go, and that's down'. The pressures of his career, and his experiences in Europe during the War, took their toll. Toby started drinking until it spiralled out of control. He didn't go into quite so much detail at this point, and I gathered it must have been painful for him, but suffice to say he was where he was at, because of the drink.

To most, he would have been avoided, with people crossing the street so they wouldn't have to get near to him. I was fascinated by him, to think, that somebody could have attained the height that he did, then sink to depths to which he now sat. I felt incredibly sad and sorry for him. But he had a very philosophical view about life. He once asked me the question of just who in the world was the richest man? I of course, went through the usual list of expected actors and musicians, with a declining shake of the head at everyone. And upon my exhaustion of answers he told me. 'He who can awaken, get himself up, dress himself and make himself a cup of tea. He is the richest man in the world.' It took a while to understand this, and at first I didn't. Then several months later it struck me. And to this day I am humbled by this man's wisdom and simplicity. It is not our possessions that make us rich, but having health and ability is wealth indeed.

Toby entertained us with his stories of staying on the bus after its last stop, and hiding on the top deck as the driver parked up for the night in the depot, so he could have somewhere warmer to sleep than the outdoors. Of the generosity of people who would give him food and money in his hour of need. And how privileged he was to have had the opportunity to live on the side of the canal and watch the sun rise and set, albeit from under a cardboard house with perhaps an old blanket. Of course the reality for this poor man, had been bitter winters, little to no food, poor health and no physical comforts. And yet, he still found something wonderful in everything he encountered. Floydy and me couldn't help being touched by this man, who insisted on putting into our bucket this 2p coin. We used to wonder where he'd go for the rest of the day until we saw him again. And even now, I still think of Toby, a forgotten hero and master of the courtroom who fell to the evils of drink.

Floydy had the 'gift of the gab', and loved to chat to everyone, especially the ladies, and in particular the pretty ones. And they responded accordingly, clearly flattered. They'd give him their phone numbers; not the odd one, but dozens over the time we were there. I was always puzzled how he did it, and asked him his secret. He'd say things like, "tell 'em what they want to hear", or "experience lad. Just experience. One day you'll understand."

In March 1990, as the temperatures were thinking about getting warmer, and the light stayed longer into the evenings, the dispute reached a resolution. The Unions seemed powerless as the morale of the blokes declined, until a final offer was put on the table and we accepted it. Ironically what had been put in front of us at the start but which we rejected in favour of attaining something better. So, six months without pay, six months without pension contributions, and six months of standing in the bitter cold, and here we were as a mob of workers, broken by the Thatcher Government. I'd done alright, and without a mortgage and still living at home, the experience was a bit of excitement. But the novelty had worn off and I, like most was bloody glad to get back to work.

Our last union meeting before the return to work coincided with Floyd's 65th birthday and the eve of his retirement. One of the ambulance control girls and myself decided that we couldn't let the occasion go by without something for the old boy to remember. We arranged everything a few days before the meeting and put the chairman of the meet in the picture. The day arrived and all the blokes and girls amassed in the mess room at Henrietta Street. The room was packed with over a hundred people, crammed in, some sitting on the window sills that overlooked the pavement outside, and others standing around eagerly awaiting news of our impending return to work. Little did they realise what they were about to witness.

I have a terrible habit of laughing at the wrong moment, and giving things away, so along with a few late comers, I stood in the doorway where I could hide my face but equally see everything, including Floydy. The meeting started with a serious tone, and the confirmation that the dispute was over, and that a return to work was ear marked for a few days time. There was a huge sigh of relief from most of us, for perhaps different reasons; many had fallen behind with their rents and mortgage payments, and the bailiffs and debt collectors had long since been rattling their doors. And then there were the plain bored who could see no sense in fighting for something which was never in our reach to start with.

After half an hour or so, most of what needed to be said, had been discussed, and I could see the guys becoming fidgety. Chairs started to scrape the floor and clearly, Floydy sensed the meeting was coming to a close, by putting his jacket on. Taking out a box of cigars from his inside pocket, he opened the box and stuck one in the corner of his mouth before striking a match and puffing on it to produce large plumes of smoke before finally drawing for slightly longer, inhaling, then blowing out another batch of cigar smoke with some satisfaction.

Before anyone had actually left the room, a female police officer appeared from the corridor and stepped into the open doorway, standing alongside me, knocking on the door as she did so, but not waiting for a reply, she stepped into the room with some purpose. She approached the top table with her back to the audience.

"I'm sorry to interrupt the meeting, but I'm after a Floyd Peterson whom I'm seeking to help me with my enquiries. Is he here?" The chairman pointed over her left shoulder, then stared directly at Floydy.

"Yeah, he's here WPC. Over there". A hundred pairs of eyes were now on Floydy, and his face became one of fear and puzzlement. Quickly scanning the room, it was obvious that most, if not all, looked upon the police presence as being genuine. She continued.

"Do you own a blue Ford Fiesta registration number C246 HON?" The fear came out in his reply and he stuttered.

"Err....yes.......... officer. What's the problem?" Now in order to make our plans more believable, some weeks before Floydy had told me in the mess room that he'd inadvertently let his car tax run out by mistake and had discovered his lapse some days later whereupon he went straight to the post office and re taxed it. But of course he'd been driving the car un taxed for those few days without realising. I pulled his leg about being caught by the police, to which he said that was not the case as he'd now made amends and hadn't been stopped and caught. Clearly standing in front of the woman police constable, and with the recent tax issue on his mind, Floydy must have made a connection, and went into a sort of nervous 'lets see if I can talk my way out'. He cleared his throat,

"Ermmm.....if this is about my tax, I can explain officer. You see....." She didn't let him finish.

"Come and sit on this chair", pointing to a chair she dragged in front of the top table and which now pointed towards the crowd. Floydy did as he was told, and sat. She removed her hat and then seductively, the pin holding her bob in place and down came her long hair, as she flicked her head from side to side. Her disguise was thwarted, as Floydy's face became a picture that painted a thousand words; relief, brief annoyance, then big smiles and the odd expletive. The crowd went mad as the cheering started, and wolf whistles abounded from every angle, as the 'wpc' became less and less clothed, finalising in nothing more than a G string, with Floydy's face buried deep in her cleavage.

It had been a fantastic end to the day, and to the long career of an icon. The 'celebration' was the finale of six months worth of no work, little money, total uncertainty and a reducing morale. We were cold and tired and had lost the fight, that just a few months before had been something we were destined to win. But the unions had underestimated management's determination. Maggie Thatcher beat the miners, and she wasn't about to give in to the ambos. So the stripper allowed us to let our hair down, so to speak, and celebrate seeing the back of all the nonsense of the past few months; to make a fresh start and move forward. I was particularly glad to get back to work, because I knew within months, I'd be on my 'six week' course, the one needed to move up onto 'front line'.

By the time I decided to finally start writing this book, over twenty years had gone by. I'd often thought about Floyd, and wondered how he was. Being in occasional touch with Len Crisp, graced me with snippets of news about him. First off he was still going, but had suffered a heart attack some years before, and still living in Birmingham with his wife, but that he was doing ok. But he'd be well into his eighties by now and I imagined him looking so, being somewhat immobile.

In August 2014, while on a trip to The UK, I had decided one sunny week day morning to venture into the city centre with my daughter Chloe. After parading many of the stores, we happened upon a coffee shop whereupon, after ordering some refreshment we sat at a table to eat and drink, and after doing so, we got up to go. A man stepped across my path, and I looked up. It was Floydy.

"Fuck me Bradbury, me and Karen have been sat over there looking over at you for the past 20 minutes trying to decide if it was you or not. Bald and looking right old I see, but it's definitely you. How the bloody 'ell are ya?"

For a second I was dumb struck. Here, in front of me, was a man who'd shaped me, influenced me, and taught me. Here was a true legend, who in the space of a second, invoked incredible memories of which I longed to return to. The Friday late shifts, Floyd and Kel, the sliding door Ford Transits, entrapment car crashes, the blood, the guts the gore. And of course, the laughs. I looked him in the eye and reached out a hand. He hadn't changed one bit. Not one. He still had the same look about him, and the same wicked smile. I had to stop myself from asking if he was really still alive.

"Bloody hell, hello Floyd, you look great. I can't believe it". I shook his hand firmly and with some perseverance, still stuck for words.

We chatted for about 20 minutes. He was enjoying his retirement and the two of them regularly went over to Malaysia, where he was stationed during his army days. He often talked about what he used to get up to in the army and clearly loved every minute of it and I decided he was reliving his past, not wanting to let go of the memories, much as I didn't want to either. I found myself recounting a couple of jobs we'd done but his face told me he wasn't remembering the case.

We vowed to keep in touch via email, as the time came that we had to go our separate ways. I tried to tell my 13 year old daughter about Floydy, but clearly her focus was on handbags and nail extensions. The memories were mine. And only mine.

CHAPTER 11. ACHIEVING THE STATUS.

We were all glad to get back to work, and within a few months, the dispute was becoming a distant memory. Spring had replaced winter, and the weather was warming up with the blossom showing its face and the bees developing a buzz in their step. Life at Henrietta Street was pretty much back to normal with the front line guys doing their thing, and us out patient drivers doing ours. But things were about to change for me. In the summer of 1990, I received the letter I'd waited 3 years for; a place on a '6 week Millar' front line course. My ticket to move towards the place I wanted to be; at the forefront of the emergency frontline. Being in the thick of blood, guts, gore and everything involving death and destruction where rather than being an onlooker, I would be making the decisions, and it would be me managing people whose life dangled in the breeze between living and dying.

The course started and finished, and as courses go I enjoyed it, learning all about how to be an emergency ambulanceman. It was pretty full on with the associated 'pass or fail' examinations, practical scenario training and getting used to all the different pieces of kit that adorn the rear of an ambulance. What I didn't realise at the time was that the course didn't give me reality. It didn't give me the tools to cope with the emotional and mental stresses I was about to undergo. And it didn't give me the ability to deal with working shifts and the unmentioned issues they would present, of working 7 nights on the bounce and still being expected to perform the same at the end of the 7th shift, as I would at the beginning of the first. Applying bandages to a fellow students head, arms and legs, with the associated humour that the classroom generated, was worlds apart from attending a real patient who had fallen through a plate glass door and now had an arterial bleed spurting all over the ceiling. But I developed close friendships with people who would go on to watch my back, and I theirs, sharing dangerous situations of disarming knife wielding assailants and calming irate situations, destined to get out of hand. These would be mates that would share the sight of looking down the barrels of a gun.

After successful completion of the course, I was sent on an emergency driving course; imagine a 24 year old, into his cars and driving, being put behind the wheel of a high powered car for 3 weeks of driving at speeds I'd not thought possible. Learning to negotiate bends correctly and execute overtakes safely, to make rapid progress and prepare me for the Birmingham traffic. Throwing the car around a skid pan taught me the skills and gave me the real life experience of handling skids and bringing the vehicle back under control when things got out of hand.

The course finished on the Friday, and I was re-labelled as an 80% ambulanceman; a trainee front line worker, who would receive 80% of an emergency workers wage. I felt like a dog with two dicks; I'd achieved something and for the first time I *was* somebody. Not a number anymore, but a professional, whose role would be seen as heroic and upstanding. I didn't stop to understand that this image requires experience and lots of hard work, neither of which I had achieved at this stage. And the grim reality of what I'd started, set in very quickly.

Less than 24 hours after my training finished, I started a night shift at Henrietta Street Ambulance Station, and within five minutes was on my first job, a road traffic accident, or RTA, in Hockley, Birmingham, involving a two-car head on collision, one of which had entered a duel carriageway on the wrong side of the central reservation.

The yellow shroud of the street lighting lit the arena up before me like some weird stage show, intermingled with hoards of flashing blue beacons. But this wasn't entertainment; My colleague Judy, normally seen sitting in the mess room humming to the click of her knitting needles, was now in explosive work mode. She was driving on this shift, and upon arriving on scene, was out of the sliding door of the ambulance before it had come to a complete halt. I turned to ask what she wanted me to do as she disappeared from my peripheral vision and was gone, leaving me to cope all alone with my fiery baptism. I stepped from the ambulance without a clue of what I was going to do and at that point, all my training evaded me. Opened mouthed and standing still, my hand still on the door handle of the ambulance, I gazed at what was presented before me.

The force of the impact of these two metal boxes had been devastating, and I still have a vivid memory of the carnage that was being imprinted on my inexperienced, weak feeble brain. A complete engine from a silver car, had been ripped from its mountings and hurled up the road landing some 40 feet from the remainder of the vehicle. The driver's door was missing and lay scattered among other debris on the road, and the hole it left revealed the drivers upper body, sandwiched tightly between the seat and the dashboard. I couldn't see the steering wheel but his head was slumped down, motionless, with a trickle of sticky, congealing blood dripping from his chin. Below his chest was a mangled, distorted mix of metal and clothing, with the sole of his left foot facing out and his toes pointing up in a completely unnatural position. His shoe was half the width it should have been, crushed as if in a vice, and his right hand, too was in a position only severe arm fractures would allow.

The other car was a red saloon pointing away from the city and some fifty feet from the other. It puzzled me why no one seemed to be around it, with the hive of activity being with the trapped driver of the other car. I walked towards this red car, all alone trying to think what to do. I was aware of a gathering of onlookers and I wanted them to think I knew what I was doing, but the reality was somewhat different. I was shitting myself.

I peered in through the open rear window, and at once realised how unprepared I was for this. There had been two males in the back of the car, and upon impact they'd been submarined under the front seats. Their torsos crushed into a space far too small for a body. Feet appeared in anatomical places they shouldn't have been. Faces weren't visible, but clumps of hair mixed with congealing blood and shreds of clothing were pressed against the floor of the back of the car, the front seats ripped from their mountings and combined with distorted metal, glass and tools that five minutes before had been in the boot. The driver was impaled on the steering column, as the force drove it back towards him, trapping him violently, and the steering wheel was bent beyond recognition, twisted by the rib cage of this once young man. His face was distorted with his tongue partly out of his mouth and his face blown, swollen and purple from the sheer pressure his chest had been subjected to. Death had been quick.

The front seat passenger had been ejected from the impact and had landed on the central reservation face up. He was another young bloke, probably about my age and visually, his limbs seemed straight. I checked for a pulse but there was none, and I remember asking myself if it was there but in my panic I couldn't find it? I decided to do some CPR on him. The manikins we'd practised on were so much harder than this guy whose chest felt like jelly. I pushed down on the centre of it and could feel my outstretched arms going much further down than I'd expected. I soon realised this wasn't right just as Judy appeared to my right.

"What the blazin' fuck are you doing?" She was pissed with me and red faced from being in 'go' mode. I started a reply.

"Errr, I'm ....ummm...."

"Well leave him the fuck alone, he's dead! You stupid or somethin'?"

Now it became a little clearer. This was the reason no one was with the red car. They were all gone. And very obviously so. The experience of the guys I was working with had pronounced death on them all, merely by walking past. I had so much to learn, and realised that even having done my Millars emergency front line course, I was still a grub, still the lowest of the low, and still the one who should make the tea. but I was still one rung higher than I had been, and despite being a baptism of fire, that first job didn't deter me. In fact it started to feed my hunger.

CHAPTER 12. MESS ROOM BANTER

Having now got to work on front line, I was allocated to C shift along with a good friend of mine, Carl Hart. One member of C shift was Leonard. An academic man with good taste and an incredibly dry sense of humour that I found very intimidating to start with. I always felt I was being watched and judged by him and in the early days realised I could never meet his standards, although he'd never say as such. But I knew. As time went on and my experience and abilities grew, I felt less and less like this about Len, and as he saw me makes less cock ups he became softer at the edges, and I warmed to him. I started to find him incredibly funny, and frequently would be found in fits of laughter at something he'd said but actually didn't find amusing himself. Len was such a good all rounder too. He enjoyed painting, classical music, and the culinary arts, being able to rustle up a fantastic curry in an instant. And as an author he inspired me to pen my memoirs and experiences. He was also pedantic and incredibly so when it came to cups of tea. So much so, that when Carl and I began our very first shift with them, he decided a lesson was in order if the new boys were to be making the brew.

I stood in front of the urn, alongside my nervous colleague. We felt like the school boys standing outside of the headmasters office waiting for the cane, for these were still the days of deep regard and even deeper respect for those with plenty of experience that we so obviously lacked. Len started in his soft

Scottish accent.

"Ok, now you've won the first prize and landed the top slots with C shift, we need to go through you two making a decent cup of tea. If it's not right, you'll do it again." He didn't have the regimental sergeant major about him, but this was definitely a teacher-pupil relationship, and in the eyes of the psychologists our chat was somewhat adult-child orientated. We nodded when we understood, and spoke when we were spoken to.

"Right, first off, the water must be boiling and a small amount goes into the pot to warm it. I cannot stand tea poured at the wrong temperature". He had a stern look on his face as he peered down and hesitated the point. Clearly tea poured too cool would attract criminal proceedings or something.

"So while that's warming, prepare the cups. Unfortunately, I have to put up with mugs here. These buffoons you'll be working with don't understand the bone china issue. And anyway I'm not bringing my best in to be broken by them lot." Len kept his stare at us and pointed his face towards the shift blokes. A couple of them in the mess room lowered their papers and peered over the top and through into the kitchen with a disapproving look.

"So I've relented and will allow you to use mugs. Put in a splash of milk, then empty the water from the tea pot. Put in one bag per cup, which'll be 8 if we're all in, then fill the pot to the top. Leave it exactly.....and I mean exactly 3 minutes. Stir for four revolutions clockwise and pour. I'd have you use fresh tea leaves and a strainer but it'd be more trouble than it's worth if I ingested any stray leaves. Any questions?"

I felt seriously nervous. More nervous than sitting my final exams in training school. We remained silent as we ingested all the information. I'd made tea thousands of times before of course, and it was like falling off a log. But now it had to be done to exacting standards.

Len had us make several pots before he was happy that we could be let loose with the urn. Carl was scolded (not literally) for stirring in the wrong direction, and I for pouring too soon. But I felt worthy of the shift now I had my new found skills. Of course, true to Len's superb form, it was only revealed many years later, that the tea making lesson was all done for his dry sense of humour and nothing more. Something which still makes me laugh today.

Flatulence, or farting, is something we all experience. In today's environment there is a time and place, and it is generally carried out in privacy. The 80's ambulance mess room was a predominantly male environment and farting loudly with exaggeration was seen as masculine and funny to the giver of such but as was usual, the smell put forth was seen as very distasteful and disgusting giving rise to contorted facial expressions and often a rapid leaving of the environment for enough time for the air to clear, sometimes about 20 minutes.

Of course, the farting issue wasn't carried out by all. Many had much higher standards and morals, and many were ex military where impression and decorum were very important to them. However, of those who partook in the overt bodily function, Sid from the workshops was particularly good. We won't call him a mechanic but Sid was known as Sid the hammer, on account that he would fix most things with a ball pein hammer. I recall breaking down on an out patient ambulance and Sid coming out with absolutely no tools but a hammer. The vehicle wouldn't start and after rummaging around under the bonnet, and the cursory 'whack, whack' with the aforementioned tool, the motor started as good as gold, and we had no more trouble.

Sid was renowned for producing the worst smelling flatulence. His favourite trick would be to save it all up, sidle into the mess room, lean up against the snooker table casually with his arms folded, and let a 'silent but deadly' go then sidle out again, like the silent assassin. We all got wise to him and when he appeared in the mess room, we'd all disappear.

Len too, was on a par in this department. Intelligent, artistic, well read, and the last person you'd expect to exemplify the 'art' as he referred to it, of passing wind. Len, like Sid could also clear a room, particularly if he'd been drinking copious amounts of beer the previous night. One thing no one likes to do is smell the flatulence of another. There is something particularly distasteful about the odour of gas that's been in someone's bowel, now occupying one's nasal cavity, but ironically we don't mind the smell of our own do we? Len stood in Sid's farting position up against the snooker table and let forth something poisonous, something wholly toxic and which sat there lingering like a mustard gas cloud. And as soon as he'd expelled this vile creation he moved and within seconds Sid sidled in, doing exactly the same in the self same spot, at which point he got wind (pardoning the pun) of the smell and assuming it all his own, sniffed loud and long to really fill his lungs.

" Ahhhhhh……..pure nectar".

Len by this time was smirking. This was the equivalent of anyone else laughing so hard they'd collapse, such was Len's way. He came over to me and unable to stop himself sharing the moment, told me what had happened, at the point I was retreating from the mess room, such was the odorous smell. I have a memory of Sid standing there, arms up in the air, embracing the smell he thought was his and being proud, like the carpenter having created a beautiful piece of furniture. Perhaps, this chapter to some is more disgusting than funny. Maybe. But it epitomises the times and the environment within the ambulance service at that point. I think if I'd been in that mess room for the first time at my current age and position in life, I may well have been disgusted. And as humorous as it was at the time, being in ambulance station mess rooms in modern times and being met with only clean habits and intellect is much more preferable.

The male environment of the ambulance service, as with other emergency services including the prisons, attracted a fair share of lesbians who in an apparent attempt to seek comparison with their male counterparts would adorn in crew cuts and Doc Martin boots, and were bloody awesome to work with. Out patient drivers such as myself were seen by some as being the lowest of the low by many of the blokes. But not by these girls who were always good to me and when I got onto the front line, would demonstrate their often superior working styles. Great communicators, they were passionate and humanistic with the female patients, on a par with the male patients, and didn't take shit from anybody. I worked with many of them over the years and enjoyed the experience every time.

CHAPTER 13. A DANGEROUS GAME.

Things were progressing well for me. Still hugely inexperienced and probably fairly incompetent, but I felt good about things. My enthusiasm for the job was growing, and I loved every minute. I looked forward to starting work and didn't want the shifts to end. Each job and every patient brought something new to the table; a disease I'd never heard of, or an experience that took me by surprise. Or I'd see a procedure at the casualty department that gripped me with fascination.

I'd been allocated to work a 1000hrs to 1800hrs shift with Bobby Crabb. Bob was a lovely bloke with a stable mind and attitude. He never got wound up or angry and had a great sense of humour. I warmed to him early as he treated me as one of the team and was a fantastic mentor and teacher. An ambulance veteran of some 30 years, he was a staunch union leader and had gotten many a member off the hook. So all the blokes thought highly of him.

We'd dropped off a patient at the casualty department. Bob was inside the hospital chatting with reception staff and I was tidying up in the rear of our truck as was customary of my position as the youngster. With my back to the rear of the ambulance, doors open, I became aware of an approaching vehicle with a roaring engine and a fair turn of speed. I turned around to see what commotion was about to begin to see a vehicle come skidding to halt behind the ambulance, where upon the drivers door opened and an excited middle-aged man with a dishevelled jumper and a big mop of hair started randomly shouting for help. Seeing into the back of the ambulance, he aimed his instruction in my direction as there were a few other people around. His demeanour had become almost aggressive and he was shouting for help.

At this time of my career having several months of experience under my belt I had a minor degree of confidence and as a result I did not feel out of place approaching this man and his vehicle to find out what the issue was. It was clear that his aggressive mannerism was not anger aimed at me, but rather a cry for help for somebody else who was clearly on the backseat of the car, which I saw as I approached. Stepping down from the ambulance I walked towards the car giving a cursory glance to my right and through the window into the casualty department where it was clear that the staff inside had also heard the commotion and were looking in my direction as to what the issue was. The driver had already opened the rear door of the car upon my approach and I looked in to see a young scruffy male lying motionless on the rear seat face up with his eyes half open. He looked to be in his mid-20s and wore a pair of dirty jeans, big workman-type boots and the remnants of a woolly jumper. I say remnants, because in the centre of his chest was a large scattered wound; a mix of wool, blood, hair and skin tissue with a fair degree of blood soaked both into his clothing and adorning his face. Copious amounts of blood was smeared across the back of the seats and inside of the door cards, and it was clear to me that he was both unconscious and not breathing.

I averted my gaze from the car to the open entrance of the casualty department where Bob and several nurses were quickly walking in my direction. I shouted to them to bring a hospital trolley and proceeded to grab this poor man's legs and pull him in my direction ready for when the trolley arrived.

Now standing at my side, Bob gave me a hand and between us we lifted him onto the trolley. I asked the other man as we were rapidly pushing the patient in the direction of the casualty department, what had gone on. He appeared now less excited and with a hint of confusion stated that there had been an argument and that the patient had been shot. From this point on, my concentration and that of the staff assisting with this poor unfortunate, lay in getting him into the resuscitation room.

Like a well oiled team, the nurses started cutting off his clothes whilst the consultant Doctor, who now arrived, started his assessment. It was clear to all that the patient was not breathing and was in cardiac arrest, so I started CPR. Removal of his clothing revealed a wound to the centre of his chest which resembled the top of a pepper pot spread over the entire surface. Multiple small blooded holes with blackened edges spread across his chest. There was a large area where a deep hole appeared to have blown part of his flesh away and the whole thing looked like someone had attacked him with a mincer. It was clear that this man had been shot at fairly close range with a shotgun.

Matthew, the Doctor, rapidly asked for a thoracotomy set and within seconds it's arrival saw him wielding a scalpel which was used to good effect to open this patient up from his chin to the base of his sternum, and before long a mediaeval looking device was used to cut his sternum and prise open his ribs revealing the inside of his chest cavity. It was at this point that Matthew's haste slowed to a stop and both his hands came up to indicate to all that this man was beyond help. His intentions had been to try to perform internal cardiac massage, the process of physically squeezing the heart back-and-forth in an attempt to get blood moving around the body. However, the patient's heart had been blown to pieces and was full of holes and even in my inexperience it was obvious that he was deceased.

To others involved in this scenario, this had appeared to be an unusual procedure, but not one worthy of being scrutinised. However, the scene in front of me caused mass fascination and I stood there mesmerised at what lay before me. Here was a human being cut open, and with a feeling of a post mortal examination, I was grateful to have Matthew give me a lesson in anatomy of the parts that I was seeing. It amazed me just how big the lungs were and how relatively small the heart was. I'd always assumed it was the other way around. Congealing blood filled the thoracic cavity and everything remained motionless.

This had been a thrilling experience. Very few paramedics get to see an open thoracotomy, and yet I had seen two within my first year of working on the frontline. Good or bad, it certainly predicted my future in trauma.

We'd explained to ambulance control the reason for our delay at the hospital, and then proceeded back to station to get a bite to eat.

A couple of routine cases saw the next few hours go by and then we got a call to attend a private address in Newtown, an inner city suburb with an uneasy feel about it, for a welfare check on a young female. The call had been made by her mother, who stated during the call that her seven year old daughter had been staying at the girl's dad's house for a few days but contact had not been made and the mother was getting concerned. These type of calls are frequent within the ambulance service and usually turn out to be harmless. In today's circumstances modern mobile phones are often switched onto silent or have flat batteries causing contact issues, however in the early 90s, landline based phones were the only ones in use and in this instance the mother had called and called and the phone had not been answered. As she lived some distance away, she asked the ambulance service to check on the welfare of her daughter. The mother had stated to the emergency operator that the father had a very violent history, but for whatever reason this information was not passed on to us as the ambulance crew.

I was attending, with Bob driving, and we pulled up outside of the house, a modest council type with three floors and a garage that stuck out from the front. As was so typical of the time and the place, the topography made way for an unkempt front garden with long grass, and car parts strewn all around, with an old sofa adorning the front driveway.

Everything looked quiet and there was no one about. Bob said I should ring the door bell and he'd go and look around at the rear of the property, so alighting the vehicle, we set towards our respective roles with casual nuance that dad and daughter were probably visiting the zoo or riding bikes in the park. I walked towards the front door and rang the bell but wasn't able to hear it making a noise from inside. I pushed the button again and still nothing. I rattled the letter box loudly several times and waited. Bob by now was out of sight and sound somewhere around the back of the house. I rattled the letterbox a second time and called out.

"Hello. Anyone at home?" Still no reply. It was at this point that I became aware of distant but approaching sirens, but didn't connect them to our case. They got louder. Then louder still. Then two police cars turned into the end of the road. I turned away from the house to see where they might be going, and behind me I heard a noise coming from the inside of the front door; bolts being slid back and a clear intention of the door to open. I turned around and stepped back slightly to politely engage with the house holder and ask him if everything was OK. The door opened, and to my horror, there stood an aggressive looking bloke with a machete in one hand and a carving knife in the other. My eyes opened wide and instinctively I quickly stepped back further with an intent to leg it away. The armed bloke rushed forward and swung the knife at me as the sirens got louder still and police cars came skidding to a halt right outside of the house. We caught each other's eyes and he shouted.

"I'm gonna fuckin' kill ya". He furthered himself in my direction, but by now one of the police officers, baton drawn and running towards us shouted back at him.

'PUT THE KNIVES DOWN. PUT THEM DOWN. NOW". This appeared to startle the bloke who looked around him, then threw both weapons on the roof of the single storey garage at the front of the house. I, meanwhile was retreating backwards towards the ambulance. Bob then appeared and having realised what had gone on, also made towards the ambulance drivers side, and the both of us got into more relative safety. The man by this time had disappeared back into the house, and within seconds more police cars screeched up the address.

It transpired that when the original call had come in, the police were notified of the address and several red flags of violence attached to it and were attending for our safety. Part way to the scene however, the male at the house had called the police directly to say that he was holding his young daughter hostage with weapons, following a heated argument he'd had with his ex-partner, the lady who made the initial call to the ambulance service requesting a welfare check. Somehow, Bob and myself had not been party to any of this and had assumed a safe and cozy job, with all to be found fine, and a return to station for a cuppa.

We sat in the front of the ambulance with me barely able to comprehend what had just happened and how near I had been to severe injury if not death. Bob of course was not aware of the weaponry that I had been threatened with only the arrival of the police and was wondering what all the fuss was over. The police stood at the foot of the drive some 20 feet from the front door attempting to talk to the male inside. The door of course was shut.

Suddenly, I heard a loud crack and a pop, and instantly there was a small hole in the top of the windscreen. I looked up at an upstairs window and could see the man pointing a rifle from an open window in our direction. Bob turned the ignition key and although the vehicle started straight away that momentary lapse before it did made me expect the arrival of another bullet. He selected reverse gear and we rapidly went backwards away from the house. The police had also taken refuge behind their vehicles and now were shouting at the house for the man to throw his weapons out of the window. It was clear from the noise and what I could see from our vantage point that the man was smashing the house up inside.

More police cars turned up, including a dog van and the scene resembled a major incident with neighbours coming out to see what all the noise and fuss was about.

Amid the chaos, the front door of the house opened slightly, and the man stood there holding the collar of a Rottweiler dog which he lurched forwards in the direction of the police and shouting, "kill". The dog, however, had ideas of his own and wandered onto the drive in no particular direction as if this was his chance to go for a walk and have a sniff around. He approached a lamp post and lifted his leg up against it to have a piss, then sauntered off. By now we were parked several houses down from the address, sitting and waiting while the stand off proceeded. The police seemed to have the situation as an ongoing one, and we were there probably for the male householder, after the police would go in, full riot gear a blazing, to drag him out, in the event he would receive injuries. I was still quite excitable following my experiences but Bob, in his usual style was calm and collected, as if he were waiting at a queue to buy petrol. Neither of us were injured, but as far as I was concerned that was more by luck than judgement.

We sat there for what seemed like a fair while and nothing seemed to progress. He was still inside, behind a locked front door and the police were still talking to him from the garden but had made some progress by a rifle having been thrown out of an upstairs window. The Rottweiler dog made a reappearance from his travels and stood in the road as if he didn't have a care, revelling in his new found freedom. Now there are times in life where we all look back and wish we could reverse time, so that an event that has taken place, can be negated. Hindsight is indeed a wonderful thing. In his infinite wisdom, Bob decided that the dog needed to be chained up so it could be out of harm's way. So he alighted the ambulance and asked a nosey neighbour for a length of rope, where upon, holding said rope approached the dog to tie it up. The fact that a police dog handler was on scene mattered not. The dog of course, was having none of it, and as Bob fronted up, the dog proceeded to launch at Bob's left arm, hanging on to the upper part like his life depended on it, and shaking Bob like a rag doll before eventually letting go. Clearly shaken and injured, Bob approached the back of the ambulance where I'd now opened the doors, and climbed inside, sitting on the stretcher with blood pouring off his dangling hand, his uniform coat rather torn, and a grimace on his face that exuded his pain.

I removed his coat to be met with a severely torn bicep muscle and an arterial bleed. The wound was hosing out and spraying blood. In these circumstances the old adage of position, expose, elevate, pressure worked well and before long, Bob was laid out on the stretcher, top half clothing removed, with his arm sticking straight up in the air, and me applying pressure from a large field dressing. I wrapped several more around the wound and the bleeding seemed to stem, although Bob was clearly in excruciating pain. For now, my colleague was the patient and I drove him into the General Hospital and left the hostage situation to deal with itself.

Bob underwent surgery and made a good recovery. The young girl was found at a different address and the house was then stormed by police who took the male into custody and he was charged with a myriad of offences and went to prison. Bob was criminally compensated as the dog was used as a weapon. The ambulance windscreen was replaced and the first aid kit was restocked. Bob and I went on to receive a Chief Officer's Commendation for performance above and beyond expectation, and putting our lives on the line in the duty of helping others. This is a somewhat strange accolade. Ambulance staff do this on a frequent basis, going into risky circumstances where even dynamic risk assessments aren't enough. If we only ever entered the scene when it was 100% safe, we'd never see a patient. I've been covered in petrol, threatened with knives, spat at, shot at, punched, kicked, threatened with violence and received needle stick injuries. They shouldn't be, but alas are, part of what front line ambulance staff do. If the stories get out, we're heroes and receive an award and it gets in the papers. If no one notices, the event remains under wraps. I've even known of staff disciplined because they put themselves in harms way when maybe they shouldn't have, knowing the risk, but still did it anyway, saving the patient and getting a bollocking in the process because the health and safety director, who sits behind a desk all day, deemed the actions inappropriate.

And so ended another exciting event, that at the time, passed without much thought.

CHAPTER 14.
SAVING FACE.

In the 1980's the ambulance service was staffed by characters; total individuals whose traits were allowed to be publicly aired due to several factors. Lack of health and safety, pre I.T. and discrimination. People 'got away' with acts that would have been regarded as disciplinary in modern times. Of course much of this is a good thing now. We can rest easy knowing elements such as bullying and discrimination won't be tolerated in the workplace. But sensibility has sometimes been pushed aside by stupidity and bureaucracy. It often seems that the guys on the shop floor have no issue with some elements that go on, but management can't be seen to be ignoring some issues for fear of futuristic retribution.

In the days when men and women would sit for extended periods of time between jobs in the mess rooms, frivolity and humour played a big part. It was sometimes at an individual's expense but everyone seemed to give as good as they got. No one complained to the boss of being picked on, and tit for tat pranks were common place, as were comedians, who, one could argue, created an escape or an arena for stress reduction. In the aftermath of a several death road traffic accident, black humour had its place amongst the mugs of tea at the mess counter. Well, all except the death of a child, which became sacred and where humour never, ever played a part.

One such comedian was Rake Growler, a giant of a bloke who'd originated from Holland but had grown up in the back streets of Birmingham and as such, had a broad Brummie accent. Rake was a good ambulancemen, conscientious with his duties and full of compassion for those that genuinely needed and deserved it. But he had two traits which appeared on a regular basis; his ability to attract trouble, and his extraordinary large penis. Rarely a month would go by, where an individual, often under the guise of drink, chose unwisely to take Rake on. His motto of 'ask questions later', meant he never came out the loser. But he just seemed to attract this often unwanted attention even when he was off duty. When out walking once in the wilds of the countryside, miles from anywhere, he happened across a young man, mugging an elderly lady for her bag at gunpoint. As the lad ran towards him, clutching his haul, Rake didn't even have to chase him, merely reach out, grabbing the gun, and with one punch it was all over. For this he was given a bravery award, and although he played it down somewhat, he let everyone know for sometime after.

His actions with his penis, however, merely attracted woeful cries as he'd creep up behind an unsuspecting colleague dozing in the chair, carefully laying his appendage on their shoulder, to the initial amusement of the rest of the shift, until they became bored of the game and where it would only be played when a new shift member came along. Doris, the cleaner, was often subjected to his manhood in a joking fashion, and her response was always one of humour.

"Oi, ya dirty basted," she'd shout, with a smile on her face, and a can of Mr Sheen in her hand. "Ya want me to polish that relic?" As he'd wave it at her from across the room.
"Ya can polish this baby anytime ya like Doris. Just don't tell my missus."

One morning in the mess room, Doris was dusting the pool table and happened to be standing alongside it holding a cue upright. Rake had sidled over while she'd been distracted, and with a quick zip and a lengthy reach into the fly out came the monster laying it on the table. Before he could say anything, and without even blinking, down came the pool cue and struck Rake's penis with some force. This was probably the first and only time Rake had been truly dropped to his knees. And aside of a sort of whimper, he never said a word, merely got himself up after some considerable time, and nursing somewhat of an injured part, limped off to the gents to examine, one would have guessed, the damage. Doris stared at him throughout the whole ordeal, and never said a word. I knew Rake for some years after that, but strangely, never saw his penis again.

Another man whose penis made a regular attendance in the mess room was Bevon Ward. Bev originated from the days when ambulance drivers were little more than just that. Drivers with a first aid bag, some of whom would go the pub between jobs on the late shift. He was a strange mix of mental health and vast experience, and during his years, there was little he hadn't seen or dealt with. Military time spent in Northern Ireland, then dealing with the aftermath of the Birmingham pub bombings in 1974, had taken its toll, and Bev found himself in various psychiatric hospitals when he was particularly unwell, and bouts of duty when he wasn't. As time went on, 'Bab' as he had been known for many years, (allegedly 'baboon Bevon' due to being hung like a baboon) declined to the point, even in those days, where his actions could no longer be tolerated. Bev had a penis that was reputed to be somewhat huge, and his behaviour, as time wore on seemed to be more and more orientated around this fact.

On one occasion Bev found himself working alone on a night shift. His mate had gone sick and as often happened during those times in the 80's, Ambulance Control, known as Metro Control, wouldn't send out a single crewed vehicle for safety reasons. Bev delighted in this fact, as now he could settle down for the night, get some sleep, and see off this night shift with considerably more comfort than most. So, after the late shift had departed, Bev, now alone in the station, decided upon a celebratory 'wank' in the toilets using a 'jazz mag' from the top draw of the mess room office table as his motivation. These magazine were the ones that adorned many a male orientated environment of the era and before, and many fire and ambulance stations had them littered around. So, with a steaming mug of tea in one hand, a jazz mag in the other, and presumably erotic thoughts swinging through his mind he disappeared into the gents toilet for the aforementioned deliberation. It must be noted that the men's toilets were located off a corridor and opposite was the mess room door. At the end of this corridor was the exit door into the garage where the ambulances were parked and served as the entrance into the main building from outside.

A Short time into his pastime, the Metro phone rang. Presuming it was a job from Control which Bev knew he couldn't attend, he let it ring and carried on. But it rang, and rang, and rang and after some considerable time, Bev thought he should answer it. So, now with his cock in one hand and a soft porn magazine in the other, and with his trousers and jocks around his ankles, he shuffled out of the toilets, along the corridor and into the mess room to pick up the phone, which was still ringing.

"Hello Bev, it's Carol from Control". This was met with a suspicious grunt. What the hell does she want? Doesn't she know I'm having a wank fer fuck's sake, Bev pondered.

"Yeah, what" was his blunt reply. Carol continued….

"We're sending someone over to crew up with you. There's another solo at West Brom". This was the ultimate disappointment for Bev and his night of sleep and pleasure was now off the cards. He tutted loudly and with disapproval before rudely replying.

"Can't you send 'em somewhere else?" Apologetically, Carol

stated that she couldn't and Bev put the phone down in disgust. But he reasoned that West Brom station was miles away and the bloke coming over would be at least an hour. This perked him up a little and he shuffled back towards the toilets to complete his 'business'. Opening the mess room door and shuffling back into the corridor, Bev was met with a very young, West Bromwich female, 'green behind the ear' ambulance women. Her vision of this middle aged bloke, porno mag in left hand, trousers and pants round his ankles, huge but now flaccid cock hanging southwards to his knees left her more than shocked and very embarrassed. But in true Bev style, he just turned to her and with a confident style spoke.

"'Ello luv, I'm Bevon. Go an' put the kettle on will ya? I'll be finished in a minute." And finish off he did, with this little exercise earning him yet another written warning.

Another such occurrence happened in the mess room one morning on the early shift. The station had recently employed a new cook, a shy young girl with multi coloured spiky hair and a face full of piercings. She only worked mornings to service the culinary needs of the blokes on the early shift. So, she'd brew numerous mugs of tea and cook enough breakfast sandwiches to feed an army. A plate of sausage sandwiches was placed on the kitchen counter, being at waist height, where Bev stood, and while her back was turned, he placed his penis in one of the sandwiches, whereby the end clearly stuck out beyond the crust and onto the plate. The cook turned round, looked down at the plate, as Bev calmly spoke.

"Who's for sausage sandwiches then?"

The sound of smashing crockery signalled the dropping of several mugs of steaming tea, as she ran from the kitchen, in the direction of the gaffers office. What made it worse for the poor girl was the raucous laughter that erupted from the rest of the blokes who in the period fashion, found the event very funny. Bev, on the other hand didn't appear to be amused by it, and without cracking his face simply sat down to read the paper, with a bemused look on his face. He didn't complete that shift. Nor any others since, but was returned to room 41 in the local mental hospital....

These three ditties detract from the main theme of this chapter, but involved a sexual theme, which is what reminded me of them. As I go through my day, and think of a particular memory that I found funny, poignant or interesting, I note it down and transpose it later, and felt these formed an appropriate intro for the up and coming.....

South Capleton was then as now, a bustling community of old fashioned shops and fresh vegetable sellers on the pavement, intermingled with second-hand furniture shops bargaining with would be buyers in loud voices. Brightly coloured sari's holding the hands of little ones adorn the pavements and the smells of Indian spices fill the air. Traffic has always been bad due to parking on either side of the road, double in some places for deliveries, making traversing the route in an emergency ambulance somewhat frustrating.

Brian was a civil servant. With his grey suit, manicured beard and briefcase, he'd take the train every day to the office, returning home at 5 o'clock for his tea waiting on the table. At the weekend he'd take Margaret shopping and on Sunday you'd find him pushing the lawnmower, still wearing a shirt and tie. In his early 60's, Brian's home life was stereo typical of a near retiring government white collar worker. He was a member of his local Masons, and his wife too was held in high esteem within their local community, giving time to The Women's Guild, the Lions and other such charity work. Their son had become an accountant and had given them a couple of grand children, and their daughter had married an American politician, so with all off spring grown up and left home, Brian and Margaret had the time to become model citizens and were held in very high regard.

He was dependable and predictable, and he was the epitome of routine. Once a month he'd come to Birmingham from his home in the south for a business meeting, staying over night and travelling back the next day. Except Brian held a secret. Behind closed doors, he stepped out of his routine; out of his lifestyle, to enjoy a pastime a little less 'upstanding'. Following his meetings he would travel to Sparkhill, to a gap between the shops which led to a stair well, at the top of which was a plain door. He'd knock at precisely midday and meet with Janine for exotic, kinky sex. Here, he could live out his fantasy and his cravings, and get a service his usual hum drum lifestyle didn't even know existed. He liked it rough, and got off on being tied up, whipped and degraded before having his way with a woman who would let him do anything to her.

Janine was a prostitute whose forte was the provision of a specialised service. A somewhat 'larger framed' lady, she'd developed a clientele who sought out this type of past time and having been seeing Brian for a long time had created almost an emotional relationship with him. But don't get any misconceptions about this lady; having once held an academic, professional post she had intellect and personality, and had decided that she could earn more money to keep her young family via this means than using intellect. And every month, Brian would go back to his wife, none the wiser of his activities, falling blissfully back into the routine of a sixties couple, living a charitable and honourable lifestyle.

"Metro Eagle 3. Eagle 3 you receiving?" The dulcet tones of the radio sealed my lack of enthusiasm. We'd had a belly full of hum drum since starting at 0700 hrs, and it was now 1250hrs with station, tea and a sandwich just a distant oasis. I'd so hoped of a return to station and some refreshment.

Reluctantly, I picked up the mic and tried to sound enthusiastic. After all, it wasn't the fault of the control staff.

"Eagle 3 go ahead over".

"Eagle 3 we've got a cardiac arrest for you in South Cap when you're ready for details over....." They'd got my attention. Taking a hungry crew, desperate for a brew and something to eat and give them yet again, something which didn't warrant an emergency ambulance, and demotivation is inevitable. But give the same crew something they can get their teeth into and it's a different story. Road traffic accidents, shootings stabbings.......and cardiac arrests. Ah yes, the adrenaline, the rush, the chance to really make a difference. With a ping of excitement and adrenaline, I returned quicker this time.

"Roger go ahead over". With the address given, the blue beacons spun into life and the air horns woke up blaring at everyone around to do the same.

Negotiating the South Road was always a nightmare when on a 9's, and this was no different. Weaving the entire width of the tarmac to avoid double parked vans delivering beds, elderly Indian ladies steering slow walking frames and the sheer headache of excessive stationary traffic. In, out, to the left, up on the pavement, mind the child, pick up speed, brake hard. Ten minutes saw a slow progress of some two to three miles until we pulled up outside of the address alongside a line of parked cars. In cases such as these, inconveniencing other road users has to come second place to the safety of the patient we're attending. So abandoning the ambulance in the middle of a main arterial road, I alighted and grabbed as much kit as I could carry, as did my crew mate Jenko, and dodging the pedestrians on the pavement we made our way to a set of steps in between two shops clearly marked with the number we were looking for. I sprinted up the wooden steps and headed for the open door at the top. Jenko, in his usual manner, followed in a somewhat slower pace. I called out as I entered a kitchen type area, to be met with a woman's voice seemingly not in panic.

"In here" she said, and following the sound led me through into a back bedroom.

Desperately in need of decoration, and smelling of damp, the room contained a double bed with ruffled sheets on top, and not much else. The walls had peeling paper from a bygone era and the floor was adorned with a carpet more suited to that of a dreary pub foyer, being somewhat threadbare but clean. It's often been said that ambos have this ability to determine exactly what's gone on within the blink of an eye of entering a scene. And that's right on the mark in 99% of cases. On the floor lay a man in his 60's, semi clothed, with a grossly obese lady dressed in basque, stockings, suspenders and high heels, performing CPR on the male. Before I'd put down my gear, I'd deduced she was a prostitute, who serviced her client, beyond the knowledge of his wife, for many years, whilst up on business, and that normally, he led a very Christian and charitable life. The whole scene just had an obviousness about it.

"Hello, I'm Dave, if you're ok with continuing CPR, I'll get on with other things." Now wasn't the time for pleasantries; succinct and to the point. The woman's CPR was good. She'd done this before.

"Ok" she replied, continuing to push on his chest. "We were, well, erm, how do I say......?" She paused with some embarrassment, "well into the thick of it. Brian was ....taking me from behind, and really going for it, when he fell to one side and onto the floor. I thought he'd just lost his balance but he didn't answer me when I called his name." I half listened in my busy world being vaguely aware of a huge buxom cleavage wobbling in front of me, as Jenko entered, and sprung into life as only a cardiac arrest can provoke. Seeing the situation, and the help we had from this lady, he became the gofer (a term used to describe a 'runner' - one who fetches and carries to aid in the egress department). Zips on the cardiac defibrillator whizzed down and patches became slapped onto the chest in front of me as side defibrillator paddles came out to do their stuff. The reading showed asystole, a flat line implying no heart activity. Without the ability to shock his heart, I stuck several sticky electrodes to his chest to monitor the rhythm, and turned to his airway. She'd clearly been performing CPR for a while. Vomit adorned his face and mouth making the insertion of a tube into his airway all the more difficult. After some suction from the Laerdel unit, the tube was tied off in place and attached to a bag-valve-mask, and I could begin the process of gaining intravenous access, inserting a large bore needle into an arm vein to aid the giving of potentially life saving drugs.

My impression of the scene and goings on was now gaining impetus. The woman before me had a facial expression of multitude; intellect, intelligence, professionalism and embarrassment. Drugs went in, ventilation continued, as did chest compressions, until some time had gone by, with no change to his heart rhythm which still showed nothing. His time was up, and she knew it.

"It's hopeless isn't it" she said with a heavy heart. I detected feeling, and love, and a real care in her heart. I stopped. It was time.

"Yes, I'm sorry, it's no good. He's had the best chance possible, but he's gone". I expected tears, but they didn't come, as she also stopped and remained still for a short time along side of him, looking at the now still, half open eyed deceased male before us both, with a sorrowful look upon her face. She stepped back and sat on the edge of the bed.

"I know what you're thinking", she said. "I'm a working girl, but it's not like what you think". I'd started to warm to this lady. There was something about her that demanded understanding and almost pity.

"Hey listen", I returned, "we're not here to judge anyone. What people do in their back yard is their business". She didn't respond for what seemed like a long time, and I was just about to start thinking of something to say when she came back looking at me with more of a reminiscence of an interview candidate.

"I'm Janine by the way. I used to be a nurse, until my husband left me with two young kids and not enough means to keep them. A friend of mine had been on the game and got me into it for easier, better money."

I started to feel like an agony aunt, as she continued, while I cleaned up the patient from all the shrapnel that I'd inflicted upon him. I remained silent but attentive. She'd got to get this off her chest.

"Slowly I built up a regular clientele. Brian's been coming here for the last ten years. Every 4 weeks, without fail. He was such a sweet gentleman." She sighed. "Bringing me flowers..............he used to say to me that I'd saved his marriage. He hadn't had sex with his wife for fifteen years. And while he was seeing me, he didn't need to...." Her facial expression changed to one of concern as her forehead frowned, "does....errr, does his wife have to know? I mean, she seemed like such a lovely person. Brian used to speak of her with such love. Does she need to know?"

I pondered the question for a short time. A surreal situation sat in front of me. Here was Janine, clad in all the gear, clearly about to feature in police statements which would eventually get back to Brian's wife. I looked at Jenko, who knew what I was thinking.

"It's your call Dave".

"Janine, go change into something ordinary and everyday, and quickly before the Police get here." I said. She obeyed without questioning, probably glad to have the opportunity to get Brian 'off the hook' so to speak, and disappeared from the room. Jenko set the carry chair up and both of us knew the plan without word. Carry Brian down to the ambulance, call him deceased there and tell the police we'd picked him up from the pavement. The timing went like clockwork. Once in the back of the ambulance, Janine appeared, jumped in, kissed him and went to exit before turning to me.

"Thank you. Thank you from the bottom of my heart" she said with tears now reaching the corners of her mouth, as she jumped down from the closing doors. A minute or so later saw them re opening with the smiling face of a police officer saying hello.

"What we got then lads?" He asked as he climbed in, shutting out the prying public behind him.

"Well, it's like this officer......we had this call to a collapse on the pavement........" I started. Jenko looked away, as the policeman retrieved his notebook and started writing.

I often wondered what his widow thought about him being found some distance from where his meetings were, or if his meetings ever really took place. Perhaps she thought he was at the office during these visits. But whatever, here was a classic case of don't judge the book by the cover. Rarely have I felt pity and sorrow for someone such as Janine. They had a contract sure, but I reckon it had gone further than this. She cared for this man; the kiss on his cheek and the hand brushing up his forehead before she exited the back of the ambulance said it all. My humanism likes to think Janine gave up her 'career' after Brian's death, that she realised she was worth more than selling herself. Perhaps she was waiting for a sign to do so, and this was it. But who knows where she is now, or what she is doing?

CHAPTER 15. THE POTENTIAL ENDING OF A CAREER. PART 1

I started settling into C shift and was glad I'd been allocated there. Being in this position was a bit like when you go to secondary school and you eagerly await which house you're to be put into. It was a mixture of trepidation and fear. And on this occasion, Lady Luck had been on my side. C shift was the very same that Floydy and Kelvin had been on. Floydy of course had by this time retired, and Kel had left the service for pastures new, but there were some great blokes to work with, and alongside two other newbies fresh from training school, Big Brian and Carl, I didn't feel the odd one out. I got on well with both of them, but Carl and myself developed a lasting friendship that perhaps only develops when you've seen the worst of society, and scenes no humans should. A sort of bond where physically and psychologically, you pull each other through. A bit like soldiers do.

One of the blokes I worked with was Adam Jenkins. A well presented guy about ten years older than me. Jenko was 'one of the quiet ones', the type that normally remains subdued for most of the time but rumble him at your peril. I liked Jenko, and from the start we seemed to get along well. Although an ambo for many years, he was a newly qualified paramedic still finding his feet, and I the complete new boy, and his experience mentored me well. I worked with him for about a year, and as time went on, it was clear he was not happy in the job and increasingly resented the violence, language and hassle that alcohol brought to the party when working weekend late shifts in the city with the pubs and clubs. Every second job was drink related and unless they were merry and good humoured with their cut heads and split lips, Jenko found them more and more intolerable. I watched this polite, mild mannered professional, become angry on a steady plane downhill until he blew. And it got to the stage where many jobs we went to brought the fear of a complaint. I guess his fuse was just getting shorter.

One day in the mess room, John the Leading hand came in from the office to have a word with Jenko about his annual leave. It started off as a polite conversation. But Jenko didn't agree with John's calculations and the heat was wound up. John wasn't an arguer but was trying to get his point across. Tempers flared, then big Brian, at 6 feet 5 inches stood up to side with John. My crew mate, at just under a foot shorter than Brian jumped up and the two tables and several chairs between them were picked up and hurled across the room. Even Brian could see the aggression in Jenko, and used discretion as the better part of valour on this occasion. John quickly left the mess room, which was also probably a wise move.

Out on the road, we received a call to The Dome nightclub for an intoxicated female. The first aid room handed over to us what appeared to be an intoxicated female of about 20. She lay on her side on a mat, moaning and retching, and lying in her own vomit. She was placed onto our carry chair and taken to the ambulance, where the commotion brought her friend running out of the club door also heading for the open doors of the back of our ambulance. If there is one thing most ambos dislike more than drunk patients, it's drunk friends who often become a real headache, preventing proper clinical care from being delivered. But the aim of a good clinician is to nurture and guide both patients and friends to do what the clinician wants them to do. It's done by humour, keeping relaxed and being nice, and often they remain the same. And in this case the female friend was ok but she made the assumption of jumping of the rear of the ambulance without asking. Jenko took exception.

"And who might you be?" He asked the young lady who by now had sat down on the chair, her hair dishevelled and her make up looking a little tired, walking barefoot with her shoes in her hand. She looked at him, in the way only intoxication can do,

"I'm 'er best friend, and I'm comin' to the 'ospital wiv 'er" she slurred out.

"O are you? I don't think so. Now would you mind stepping off the back of the ambulance so we can take your friend to the hospital?" She started getting annoyed.

"But I'm 'er friend an' I wanna go to the 'ospital wiv 'er." she leaned towards her friend who by now was lying on her side with congealing vomit sticking her hair in a clump across her face, "you alright Trace?" Then she looked at Jenko again. "Is she alright mate? I reckon someone's spiked her drink, coz Trace can put away much more than she's 'ad tonight". She clearly wasn't listening to Jenko.

"Look, I'm telling you now, get off the ambulance or I'll call the police, and the longer you stay, the longer it will be before your friend receives hospital treatment". The mannerism of the pair of them was heightening. She went to shout something at him, and he launched at her, grabbing her wrist and in one swift movement, threw her off the back of the ambulance.

"I told you to get off the back, and I bloody well meant it!" How she managed to remain upright and not fall over was beyond my comprehension, especially based on how drunk she was.

My heart sank, and my thoughts turned to the complaint that was sure to ensue.

One of our regulars was Damien Rogers. His party trick was ripping an aluminium can in half, then hacking at his wrists to the worry of concerned onlookers in the city centre who would dial 999. Damien was most often aggressive, abusive and was usually intoxicated. One night shift, Jenko was driving and we got a call at about 1o'clock in the morning to report of a male slashing his wrists in the city centre. We duly attended, remaining pretty quiet en route as was the norm at that time in the morning, and we both knew who it would be. Damien was on form, but a few quietening and reassuring words from me saw him reasonably cooperative, even allowing his wounds to have dressings applied. He sat in the back of the ambulance and off we drove. But almost immediately, he started playing up, ripping off the bandages and after we'd travelled no more that half a mile or so, he stood up rushing to the rear of the saloon, and before I could grab him, he'd opened the rear doors and jumped out.

"STOP, he's jumping out the back!" The rear door violently swung back shut again as I got to it. My heart raced, as Jenko never even slowed down from the steady 25mph he'd been doing.

"Serves him fuckin' right if he gets killed" he said, with such a calm approach, I couldn't believe it. I grabbed the door and opened it, to see, to my complete amazement, Roberts, barely upright and staggering, but running into the distance. My fear of my career being cut short, rapidly changed to relief. Jenko casually continued driving as I shut the door. He got on the radio, "Metro Eagle 3, er... Our patient has declined hospital treatment, thanked us for our time and left the ambulance..." Strangely, I never saw or heard of Damien again.

Historically, for the mere fact that the rear of ambulances are 'van' like, they have been used for the carriage of anything and everything. And I'm not in the slightest referring to patients. You name it, and it's a sure bet it's been in the back of an ambo. Jack Salter moved his mother's entire house using all the blokes on his shift, during the shift. They all clocked in at 7am and each time a job came in, they'd weigh up whether to pop round to Mabel's place before venturing on to the patient, or if it seemed like a real emergency from the call, they'd leave it until after they'd cleared from the hospital, to pick up a wardrobe, a settee or a bed to take round to the new flat on route back to the station. Mabel saved on removal costs, and the guys got bacon sandwiches and mugs of tea. It was almost part of ambulance culture.

Late one chilly November evening, a routine maternity case came in to the mess room for Jenko and me. Labour had descended to Mrs Bibi and we were dispatched to Handsworth to pick her up and take her into Dudley Road Hospital maternity unit. The job was entirely non emergency and as I sat in the rear with her, the expectant mother barely had any labour pains en route, and as she didn't speak any English, the air remained pretty quiet. Jenko turned the ambulance into the entrance and drove the short road round to the maternity unit. But before we got there he pulled up short. I looked up from my paperwork after I became aware that we hadn't arrived at the unit and neither had Jenko alighted the driver's door. He was looking out of his window into the darkness, and appeared to be impressed by something he saw. After a moment, he selected first gear, and we moved forward and on to the delivery suite.

The rear doors opened and cold air rushed in as Jenko leaned forward and pulled down the step for us to walk down. As I stepped out I ushered my patient to follow and in we went for handover. It was all routine, and my partner was keen for us to get out and back to the ambulance.

"Come on", he said. "There's something I want". Intrigued, I remembered back to his momentary stop and assumed this was it, following this 'man on a mission' outside. He drove us round the corner to where there were some works in progress in an old store building. We pulled up behind a skip overflowing with rubble and empty paint tins. Jenko slid open the door, pulled up his collar against the biting cold and grabbing a torch, jumped out and walked towards the other side of the skip. Curious to have revealed to me the root of his want, I followed, and stood next to him, looking at where the light was pointing.

"What d'ya reckon?" He asked with a boyish grin on his face like he'd opened a Christmas present and discovered a top-of-the-range Scalextric set. Before me was a large metal cabinet, lying on its side and separate from a whole heap of other broken furniture and rubbish that looked like it had been cast out from the renovations but wouldn't fit in the skip. I didn't share his enthusiasm, and nonchalantly replied.

"I dunno. What is it?" He continued to look it over, but now was right into all the nooks and crannies with his flashlight, revealing cobwebs and rusty bits. He tried the handle on the door and opened it with a creak.

"It's a metal locker ya plonka. I mean, d'ya reckon it'll fit in the back o' the motor?"

The concept of misusing the resources of the ambulance service was something still fairly new to me, and being the born worrier didn't sit well with my conscience. I tried to think how I might tell him I wasn't happy to do furniture moving in case we got caught doing this sort of thing but didn't have the confidence to come out with it. So I went down the route of trying to convince him that it wouldn't fit.

"Nah Adam, it'll never fit. It's much too big. Let's leave it. Come back for it tomorrow with your brother's trailer". I preyed he'd go for it, but his determination beat me down.

"This'll be great in me shed for me gardening stuff........grab that end and give us a hand". I was suckered in and duly did as I was told. I did actually think it wouldn't fit and was relieved when presenting it to the open doors of the back of the ambulance, he agreed with me. "Bollocks, you were right".

"Ah well", I said, trying not to sound happy. "It'll go on Tony's trailer a treat". He stepped up into the rear saloon, still on his mission.

"Not bloody likely, some fucker'll have it away before then. We'll have to take the stretchers out. There's nothing else for it". My heart sank, so I tried in a last ditch attempt to get him to consider that it might actually not be dumped, and we'd be stealing it. But even that was in vain and again I found myself at the bottom end of two stretchers, removing them both and parking them up against the wall. To my disappointment, with some manoeuvring and swearing, the bloody thing went in, but the doors wouldn't shut properly. So a bandage was duly dispatched to tie the outside of the handles together.

We'd already spent about 20 minutes loading our booty, and I knew a call would soon be coming through on the radio for us asking if we were clear and available. I grabbed the mic.
"I bloody hope we don't get a job now. We're fucked if we do". Jenko had obviously sensed my total unease at the situation, and turned to look at me with a hint of annoyance in his eye.

"Your problem Bradbury, is you worry too much. We'll book clear, we won't get a job, we'll drop this off at the station and come back for the stretchers. Easy. And no one will know".

"Yeah alright then." I replied, trying to sound as if I shared his confidence, as I keyed the button on the handset, "Metro Eagle 3, now clear Dudley Road over." A quick shot of relief came in their reply. "Roger Eagle 3, return to station. Metro out."

"See!" Beamed Jenko. "I told ya you worry too much." I sat back in the chair, now experiencing some relief. Station was only five minutes away.

My relief, however, was very short lived, and the five minutes didn't come quick enough. The radio broke the silence.

"Metro Eagle 3 over". I felt a sudden panic as Comms came back to us with an assault case in the city centre. Now what the hell were we going to do? I had visions of Jenko carrying on to station, dropping off his precious metal box, then returning back to the hospital for the stretchers. This would have seriously delayed getting to our patient. Jenko remained silent for a moment after I'd written the job down, clearly deep in thought.

"This is bad timing," he said with his hands on the wheel looking through the windscreen into the darkness. "A patient won't fit in the back with the cupboard in there, but it's too far to go back to the hospital for the stretchers. Fuck it, we'll leave it here and come back for it after."

"But Jenko," I protested, "we won't have any stretchers in the back." Panic returned, but he wasn't phased. He looked me in the eye with that look I'd seen before when his feather had been ruffled.

"You have to complicate things don't you. Every situation that is so simple, you have to make difficult." He was genuinely annoyed at me, and again I was the naughty schoolboy outside the headmasters office. He continued. "It's only an assault, which means he'll be pissed, so he won't know any different." I returned the serve.

"And if he's not?" This time he turned himself completely to face me, almost as if he was squaring for a fight, and now with aggression.

"There you go again, complicating things."

He jumped out to open the back doors, and I followed. A small amount of cussing and puffing, saw a large metal cabinet sat on the pavement up against the wall of an office block. Jenko returned to the driver's seat as I looked in to the rear of our vehicle, and realised a large, empty cavern, like a disused warehouse. I shut the rear doors and once back inside contemplated, yet again, what career I might pursue when this letter of complaint came in. There was now a distinct uneasy atmosphere in the cab, as the engine revved loudly and we drove forward still in silence.

Sat on the pavement as we pulled up, was a young man with his feet crossed and sticking into the road. His head was slumped down and blood adorned the front of his once crisp white shirt that his mother had no doubt ironed, some 6 hours earlier as he prepared for his night out on the town. A trail of blooded snot linked his nose to his chest like a piece of chained jewellery. Stood behind him was a policeman, whose look told me he was glad of our arrival so he could go, and his eagerness was shown by his rapid poor handover of this pathetic chap as I alighted the ambulance. But I was still too far away to properly hear what he was saying. I caught the tail end of the sentence,

"....if he's fallen or what. There's no one else about and he ain't talking so I dunno. I gotta go." He turned and walked away, as I asked him to repeat himself, in my unconfident, quiet tone which met with silence and me trying to figure if this guy had been fighting or had merely fallen.

I knelt beside the gently snoring lad and shook him by the shoulder. "Eh mate. Wake up." With no reply I upped the volume and shook him harder, this time at arms length. Even in my inexperience, shaking a drunk sleeping man was done with some distance between us, for fear of the lashing pout that often followed their awakening. "MATE, MATE, WAKE UP, CAN YOU HEAR ME?" He stirred slightly with some mumbled noises coming from his lips, ending in the word 'fuck'. "TELL ME WHATS HAPPENED. WE'RE FROM THE AMBULANCE SERVICE". But this didn't provoke any reaction so I lifted his head a little to reveal a swollen nose and drying blood over his face. Jenko shuffled impatiently behind me with his hands in his pockets, then piped up.

"Look, he's pissed, just like I said. Let's get him loaded and we can get out've 'ere". He reached forward, grabbing our man under the arm and lifted him up. Amazingly, the guy stood, staggered and swayed and looked around him with a very puzzled look on his dishevelled and battle torn face. He looked at me through half open, lazy eyes and giggled, wafting a sickly stench of stale alcohol and cigarette breath in my direction. I quickly grabbed under his other armpit as he leaned away from Jenko and threatened to topple them both over. We walked him towards the back doors, where a step was lowered for him, and up he and I walked, into this large, empty space, which seemed cavernous without the stretchers. I heard the familiar sound of slamming doors behind me, quickly followed by the starting of the engine. Jenko was clearly still a man on a mission again, and I just about had time to get my patient laid down on the floor as we moved off. I grabbed a blanket for a pillow and one to cover him, and soon there followed the return of the soft snore as this probable result of someone's great night out slept like a baby. And within 10 minutes, we were pulling up back outside of the casualty department again, where upon the previous routine of waking our baby was repeated, and again he totally cooperated, walking down the steps and into the waiting wheelchair that Jenko had rapidly fetched in his desire to clear from the hospital quickly to retrieve his metal cabinet.

As was customary in those days, each job saw us swap roles from driver to attendant. Jenko enthusiastically jumped into the passenger seat, grabbing the mic and clearing us.

"Now, if we can just get returned to station......" His wishes were granted, and I drove us back to the spot where we would pick up Jenko's new found project. Except we didn't. Pulling up outside the office block, there was no metal cabinet. Just a pavement, littered with the previous evenings take away containers, empty cans and left overs of fried chicken and chow mein. But definitely no metal box. Jenko froze with his mouth partly open. After a few seconds he rhetorically spoke.

"This is where we left it, isn't it?" I went to confirm that it was, but he was out of the truck before a couple of my words had been spoken. He walked up and down the empty pavement as if miraculously, his prize would reappear, and his eyes would not have deceived him. But alas no. He sauntered back and climbed in. Breaking the silence after a minute. "I don't believe it," he started. "Some thieving bastard has stolen it. How could they? I'll bet it was them bleedin' travellers from Handsworth." He was distraught, like his dog had died, or his house had been burned down.

"So shall I go back and pick up our stretchers then?" I replied. He appeared in a daze.

"What.....? Er yeah, I guess so" then a glimmer of hope came across his face as he realised that maybe someone had just moved it. "Just check it's not in this alley up here in case some buggers shoved it out of the way". He pointed forwards, but as I eased it into gear and moved off slowly, a quick look down the alley as we passed it revealed still nothing. He returned to his mope, and we sat in silence driving back to pick up the stretchers. But at least I still had my job.

A few days later, we heard on the grapevine that a large metal cabinet had been stolen from the renovation works at the hospital. Apparently it had been placed by the side of the rubbish skip by mistake and had been intended to be reused. This mistake lead to the management dropping any investigation of theft. Good job really. And I, of course, said nothing.

CHAPTER 16. THE POTENTIAL ENDING OF A CAREER. PART 2

As time moved on in this first year on 'front line', my confidence grew, as did my ability. Even in those days of the early nineties, and with little more equipment than oxygen and a first aid bag, I was beginning to recognise and differentiate disease, and picked up the rudimentaries of managing them. If the patient was short of breath, they had an oxygen mask on their face. If they were in pain from a fracture, they were splinted and pain relieved with gas and air, and if they bled, they were subjected to pressure dressing and limb elevation. I started to appreciate when a patient was seriously ill or injured, and when I could take my time with a more minor issue, and developed within my own vocabulary a phrase from A.A.Milne's 'Winnie the Pooh', 'big sick' and 'little sick', and used it to determine with each patient, whether they needed urgent treatment and transport, putting the hospital on 'alert', or if they didn't.

My partnership with Jenko remained static. He still didn't seem to enthuse the job, and as such wasn't the best of mentors. Instead he duly turned up for shift, did was what needed and went home, and in the main remained quiet and calm, with the occasional flare up if someone rubbed him up the wrong way. Such was our relationship, he appeared to tolerate me and little more. Rarely did we ever speak about our home lives, and aside of knowing his wife's name and where she worked, I knew almost nothing about him. Aside that is, of his passion for gardening, which he enthused about.

One beautiful warm spring morning, Jenko and I found ourselves working a 7am to 3pm shift. It was one of those days when you could smell the freshness of the air, and hear the spring in the step of the birds busy building their nests. The daffodils were wide awake and smiling and the crocuses on the grass bank of Bristol Street proudly read the words 'Birmingham Super Prix', as advertising for the city having hosted the event a few years earlier.

Jenko had turned up for work as usual, but I'd noticed from the outset he was chirpier, brighter, and had a smile on his face, greeting me when we met at the timecard clock. We checked the vehicle, and settled back into the mess room for a cuppa. Jenko was chatty, and laughing, and when the red phone rang, he sprang up from his chair, popped his cup down and cheerily went to answer it.

"Hello, Metro...........uhhh huh. Yep. Right o.......so Dudley Road to Summerfield then? Yes that's lovely. Yes, it'll be Eagle 3. Thanks. Bye." I'd not heard him this jolly for a while, and pondered as to the cause. Now don't get me wrong, Jenko wasn't a grumpy bloke. Far from it. But neither was he normally this chirpy either. I ran out of causes of his lustre. But it was soon to become clear...

Our job was a simple routine transfer of an elderly lady who'd been to Dudley Road Hospital casualty department from her place of residence at the Elderly mentally ill unit situated at the rear of the hospital, following a fall, and now she was being returned having been discharged. We duly collected this sweet little lady, and her nurse escort, and seated them on the side facing stretchers in the back of our truck. After dropping them both off only a matter of minutes later, Jenko announced that we'd got an errand to run.

"I want to pop round to me mom's to collect a parcel", he excitedly announced, as the engine roared into life.

"Oh ok," I replied. I'd calmed a lot over the last few months and had gotten used to occasional 'errands', that took us off the beaten track. "Where does your mom live?" I enquired, taking advantage of his high spirit for a bit of chat.

"Oh not far. She's just at the top end of Handsworth. We'll go over then book clear. It won't take five minutes." I drew my seat belt and clicked it into place feeling contented as we moved forward and the heat of the sunshine hit my face through the glass.

After a short period of silence, broken only by the occasional radio transmission, Jenko piped up.

"Mom rang me yesterday, to say me parcel's arrived. I'm quite excited really cuz it'll finish a little gardening project I've got going on." I was pleased to chat like this. It was like we were proper mates; team buddies, who relied on each other. Finally, I felt I was being trusted and accepted by my crew mate and made to feel less of a newbie and a burden. I turned my gaze from the side window through to the windscreen,

"Oh yeah, what's the project?"

"Well," he enthused, "I've bin redesignin' our patio. We had some crazy paving down which looked a bit shabby, so I've taken it all up, slabbed it and put in a fish pond. But there was something missing, until the wife suggested we needed a tree to shade the pond. So I rang this mob in Coventry who advertise in me gardenin' magazine, and they do mail order plants and shrubs, so I ordered one last week and 'ad it delivered to mom's....here we are." He negotiated the ambulance to park up against the curb outside of a small house with a pretty front garden.

"You wait here," said Jenko. "I sharn't be a minute." And he alighted, shutting the door behind him, before walking up the path to the house, whereupon he opened the door and walked in.

A few moments later, Jenko's head appeared from around the side of the tall wooden back gate, which opened a small amount.

"Hey Dave? Come and give us a hand will ya?" He disappeared again and I got out of the vehicle and followed.

"Yeah, I'm coming". At the top of the path, I pushed open the gate, and walked along the side of the house and into the back garden, where upon Jenko was stood on the lawn, alongside a tree which was laid on its side. A tree through the post, I'd visualised, would be small and about three feet long. But I was slightly out with my calculations and wasn't prepared for quite what lay before me. With its roots engulfed in a large ball, I reckoned it to be about 15 feet long with a trunk at its base around six inches thick, and its tip trailing to a bendy point. It appeared that when it had started its journey from wherever it had come, it had been cocooned in a straight jacket resembling my grandad's string vest. But all that was left of it now, were a few remnants lying on the grass, as Jenko had attacked it with a pair of scissors, releasing the branches which had sprung out and stretched themselves like a waking man with arms in the air, sat on the side of the bed in the morning. I doubt Jenko could have helped himself, and must have resembled a child poised in front of a large wrapped present on Christmas morning. He now stood proudly over it, like the explorer surveying his recent discovery.

"Isn't she great?" He started. "A beautiful, healthy specimen of Elaeagnus Augustifolia. Agnes for short. Yeah. Yeah, we'll call her Agnes." But he wasn't after any form of conversation. Instead, he was in a world of his own, imagining his new found love shading his pond in the warm summer sunshine as he sat underneath it. His fantasy was cut short as he stepped back into this world as I repeated my self to him again.

"Jenko....JENKO! Is this thing gonna fit on the truck?" He snapped out of his trance and looked at me with a sense of daze.

"Errrrm yeah. Yeah, course she will. Agnes'll go right up the middle."

"Ok then, if that's what you reckon" I said beginning to share his confidence. And with no hint of my previous worries of the misuse of government vehicles, I positioned myself to pick up my end of the tree.

It was, as we'd expected, bloody heavy, as we huffed and puffed our way down the return route to the ambulance. I wondered quite how I would explain having put my back out, should it have occurred, and imagined the scenario in front of the boss. 'Well, it was like this boss. You see I was carrying this tree with Jenko......' My scenario was cut short as we reached the road and the back doors of the truck. Placing it gently back to the ground we opened the doors and contemplated just how the hell we were going to get it in. I sighed loudly, and, slightly out of breath, piped up.

"Maybe undoing that string vest wasn't such a good idea". Jenko had no option but to agree.

"Yeah, I think you're right." We both pondered for a moment, before my partner spoke. "The problem we have here, is the diameter of the branches are larger than the door opening, and they sort of point up towards the top of the tree. So the solution, is to put the root ball in first, and all the branches will follow." It seemed like a logical solution, and it meant we could leave the stretchers on the back so wouldn't have to return for them. The rooted end was fed in, and sure enough it went all the way through to between the driver and passenger seats in the front, sitting nicely in the passenger foot well. The top of the tree however, stuck out of the back door opening by about three feet, and looking inside the rear saloon, all I could see was foliage from floor to ceiling. Jenko hopped out of the driver's door, and surveyed the issue at the rear, resting his chin in his palm.

"No. It's not gonna work, is it?" He asked, already having made the decision. "It'll have to come back out, and I'll fetch it with Tonys trailer at the weekend." The prospect now, of lugging this bloody great tree back out again and all the way to where we'd picked it up from filled me with dread. But it quickly became apparent that the branches, being angled towards the top of the tree, meant that it went in far easier than it was going to come out. And I knew that Jenko's 'baby', was going to receive the utmost of care in its removal from its new temporary home. And that was going to take ages. My thoughts were cut short by the radio.

"Metro Eagle 3. Eagle 3 we have a case for you. Are you receiving over?" Now we were in trouble. 3 miles from where we should have been, and with an ambulance that wasn't in a fit state to respond. Jenko seemed as unfazed by this as he always did, but I was the first to speak.

"Hey Jenko, now, I don't worry like I used to in this sort of situation, but we could have an issue here. I mean, we don't have a motor we can respond in right now do we?" He looked at me.

"What do you mean by that?"

"Well," I said calmly, "in case it's missed your attention, our truck has got a bloody great tree in the back of it leaving no room for a patient. I mean, I can't even see the stretchers, let alone put a patient on one of them. And to top it all, we can't take it out can we?" It did vaguely cross my mind to suggest 'modifying' Agnes with a chain saw. But the thought of the chainsaw being turned on me quickly dispelled such an idea. Jenko resumed his usual 'worry free' look, then continued.

"We could always claim we've broken down, then they'll give the job to someone else.....Oh hang on though; how do we explain not being at the hospital? And Sam the mechanic's on today too. He'll see Agnes, so it's sure to get back to the boss. Well, the motor still runs, and we've done worse. I'll tie up the back doors and we'll blag it." I was wondering on what occasion we'd 'done worse', but didn't have time to argue. Blagging seemed the most sensible option in the circumstances.

Jenko gently laid the back doors up against the tree as I picked up the mic and responded to Metro Control and took down the details of our next case. A female with a cut arm. Sitting in the passenger seat, squashed up against the door making room for Agnes' root ball, I turned round to see how closed the rear doors were. And I have to admit to a twinge of anxiety when I saw a three foot gap in the doors, now prevented from opening further with a good old trusty bandage tied around the handles. I wondered if the manufacturers of these stretchy dressings ever considered just exactly what their product would end up being used for. And could sense my boss's voice in my up and coming disciplinary, including a further 'misuse of government property.' Then I remembered that our case was to Kingstanding, some 12 miles away. And all with four feet of Agnes' top sticking out the back of the ambulance. It wasn't looking healthy for us as far as I was concerned, but I had no choice but to buckle up and contemplate, yet again, what career I might next consider.....

The journey to Kingstanding, a northern suburb, was relatively uneventful. I'd wound down my window, resting my elbow out at 90 degrees, just to give me slightly more room in my cramped little space. A couple of times I turned round to look through the gap in the back doors, to see the expressions on the drivers faces who were directly behind us. They ranged from surprise, through to laughter and bewilderment, with pointing fingers and giggling children. I remained calm, still trying to suppress my growing anxiety. How on earth were we going to manage things if our patient needed to lie down on the stretcher? And then I realised I was going to have difficulty in even reaching the first aid kit, but was grateful when I realised that Jenko had already grabbed it to get the bandage that had fixed the back door issue, and placed it on the floor by the gear stick.

We finally pulled in to a cul-de-sac, and headed for the house in the far right hand corner, which as any ambulance person will know, is always the house you are looking for when in this type of road. Sure enough, the number matched the one we wanted, and I was grateful to be set free from my claustrophobic existence that I'd had to endure for the last 15 minutes. So with first aid bag in hand I pushed open the tatty wooden front gate and, dodging the old television, a car engine, several plant pots and a cat, made my way to the front door, which was slightly ajar. It was a scruffy house with a smell that only these type of houses have; a sort of musty, dirty, unclean stink that makes you want to not touch anything without wearing gloves, and wipe your feet on the way out. The sound of voices could be heard coming from inside which implied no real concern. No screams, no cries or pleas for help, and no one waiting at the road side for us waving their arms like the proverbial windmill, was a sign that this case wasn't going to be a 'big sick' one. I pushed open the door and stood to one side peering up the gloomy and smokey hallway. At the far end, I could make out a rather fat, middle aged woman leaning against a lounge chair with a tea towel wrapped around her left hand.

"Hello, ambulance", I called out.

"Er's fookin' in 'ere mate. She's 'urt really bad," came a husky male voice, followed by a coughing episode. Having steeled myself against the smell, I entered the house aware that Jenko was right behind me, hands in his pockets, looking around the walls with his mouth turned down in utter disgust. I heard him quietly speak.

"How the other half live eh? I must book a table and bring the wife to dine here..." I suppressed a laugh knowing that within two or three seconds I'd be in the lounge with our patient.

As I walked into the room, the smell intensified. It mixed with stale tobacco and body odour, and hit me aggressively as it cocktailed with the sickly heat of the gas fire. The walls were stained with brown nicotine and the whole room was cluttered with piles of dirty clothes, boxes and magazines. Cobwebs swung from every corner, and the air was thick with smoke.

The woman in front of me was about 50, grossly obese, with shoulder length, greasy dark hair, and a round, pock marked face, with what looked like remnants of her breakfast stuck to her chin. The few teeth that remained, were stained or black with rot and she wore a moustache that Borat Sagdiyev would have been proud of. Her huge, filthy, flowery dress was complimented by a hand knitted, originally lime green, I'd thought, cardigan that was clearly far too small and tight for her, gripping her upper arms and exaggerating how fat they were. Her hairy legs were oedematous, with protruding varicose veins which sat atop of blackened and dirty feet whose toes were long overdue for a visit to the chiropodist. And the odour from her was quite something, encouraging me to not get too close, as I recalled a colleague saying to me sometime before, that a wipe of Vick's Vapour menthol chest rub, placed strategically under each nostril works wonders in these circumstances. Unfortunately however, I didn't have such a luxury to hand.

She had a dirty tea towel wrapped tightly around her left hand, and the absence of any visible blood furthered my opinion that we probably wouldn't be rushing this lady into hospital with any great speed. I looked at her.

"What's your name and what's happened?" I asked with compassion.

"Fell over," she said. "I've cut me 'and. It doe 'alf 'urt."

"Ok, sit yourself down and let's have a look. Have you hurt yourself anywhere else?" I continued, as I started to unwrap the injured limb. "And tell me your name?"

"Rosemary" came the reply. "But me 'usband calls me sexy legs." The man gave a muffled laugh, and I became alarmed at the thought of......'no' I decided, 'let's not go there'.

"Ok, well, I'll call you Rosemary then." I said. The man started coughing again as he lit a cigarette. He had one final big cough then spat a huge lump of browny green frothy phlegm onto the floor in front of him, which sat there refusing to soak into the shiny filth that had once been the carpet. He drew on the fag, and over the top of his dirty glasses perched precariously on the tip of his nose, he brought his concentration once more, back to me and my actions as if nothing had happened. I momentarily stared at what I'd seen, then turned to glance at Jenko, whose eyes widened as they glanced upwards and his head turned away. I returned my attention to Rosemary, who sat down at my request. Her demeanour struck me that she wasn't the sharpest knife in the draw, and further questioning revealed that she worked a couple of hours most mornings cleaning a local shop, and that she didn't have any significant medical history and took no regular medications. This struck me as ironic given the filthy environment that she lived in, and sought of put paid to the argument that it is necessary for us all to use anti bacterial surface wipes at every occasion. I doubted she got bugs and bacterial infections any more than we did. She was not a conversationalist and seemed somewhat introverted and dominated by the much older male on the settee, as he would often answer for her.

With the dirty towel removed, the wound was revealed. A small but deep laceration to the base of her thumb that would need to be stitched in hospital. The bleeding had stopped and she seemed much more at ease now than when we had arrived. I dressed Rosemary's hand and discussed with her about taking her in. She seemed unsure but her partner convinced her it was the right thing to do, which she accepted. I turned to leave expecting Jenko to be present, but he wasn't and probably hadn't been for some time. I walked back to the ambulance and upon approach, noticed Jenko sat in the drivers seat, leaned up against the window with his arms folded and his eyes shut. I rounded towards the back doors and had a stark reminder of Agnes, who stuck out the back like it was Christmas time and we'd been and bought the station tree. Rosemary joined me at the rear and stood in silence as I untied the bandage holding the doors closed, waiting for Jenko who now stirred and made an effort to come and help. I expected my patient to say something, and waited for the question. As I opened the heavy doors to reveal an ambulance full to the brim with branches and leaves, wondering how the hell we were going to get this large lady in, she spoke.

"It's cold 'ey it?" I sighed, agreed with her for ease, took a deep breath and instructed her that I would squash the branches over to the left, allowing her to climb in and sit on the stretcher to the right. Then Jenko joined us.

"Oi! Don't damage her" he blurted out, as Rosemary climbed in, stood on some of the branches squashing the leaves, then sat down. I wasn't actually sure if Jenko's concern was aimed at me or Rosemary, but as she sat down I gently let the branches go that I'd been holding back for her, and wishing to remain at a distance, I worked my way through to the stretcher on the left and sat down. It was like being a child again and climbing a tree.....only this time in the rear saloon of an ambulance. As the rear doors were yet again bandaged to, I had to reposition my self so that I could actually see Rosemary through the foliage. She was completely unfazed by this experience, and sat in silence staring into space, occasionally adjusting her position only to find a leaf brushing across her face, or a twig sticking into her arm. She finally got comfortable, and sat with her feet on Agnes' trunk. But still she didn't ask. Jenko had one final look in his rear view mirror, clearly more concerned at his baby than us, then starting the truck, we headed for Dudley Road hospital.

Glancing through the gap at the rear, I saw the reminiscing facial expressions of humour, surprise and puzzlement, and as I couldn't actually see Rosemary now, relied on asking the occasional question of how she was, to which her reply, heard over the road noise outside, was usually that she was cold. But at least I knew she was still with us. And I wasn't particularly worried about any other crews being at the hospital and what they might think. Some of the stories I heard described almost a challenge to see who could transport the most unusual 'passenger'. A camel perhaps, or a piano.

As we pulled into the hospital, with the engine finally switched off, Jenko untied our sophisticated door closing system and after the rear step was down, he gently moved the branches over towards me to let Rosemary climb down, which she did, still in silence. I, of course, was flattened by the foliage until Jenko let go allowing me to climb out like some intrepid explorer breaking out of the thick jungle into a clearing. I instructed her to follow and inside we went, handing Rosemary over to the nurses, and saying good bye to her. And still she didn't pose the question, instead, asking me for some money for a cup of tea.

The following day, on the same shift pattern, after having dropped off at the casualty department, we went into the reception office to book our patient in. Standing there for a moment, we over heard one of the reception staff chatting to a nurse.

"She didn't half stink, and was insistent that the ambulance she came to 'ospital in had a tree growing in the back!" She put her head back and they both laughed. "You see all sorts in this job eh? Some people. I reckon she was pissed". I looked at Jenko, leaning on the work surface, feet and arms crossed. He looked at me, with a developing smile.

"Yeah, she must have been pissed eh Bradders? A bloody tree in the back of an ambulance!"

CHAPTER 17. MORE TRICKS PLAYED.

Emergency cases or 'jobs' as they were known, came to the crews in one of two ways; if the guys were on station, then via a red telephone in the mess room. As the crews came back onto station, their clip board with jobs on it would go to the bottom of the pile by the phone, and the next job that came in went to the upper most board. These days crews are rarely if ever on station, but if they are, the same principle still works; last in, last out. If they were out on the road , then their call sign alerted them to a job over the radio.

Each station in Birmingham had a call sign of a bird of prey. Sutton's was Raven, but there were Eagles, Hawks, Kestrels, Falcons etc. One of the main objectives of ambulance crews in these times was to get back to station after another crew, thereby being out last and creating longer gaps between jobs, bearing in mind that at these times there was no satellite tracking, no big brother watching you and therefore crews had an almost free reign to go wherever they wanted. Clearly Metro control, the ambulance Comms centre, then based in Dudley, West Midlands had some idea of where each vehicle was, but not their route to scene, or back to station from the hospital etc. So when one crew followed another into a hospital with a patient, they would wait for the first crew to book clear before booking clear themselves in case a job was going spare. This led to many a crew who presented the hospital with a simple case, waiting for some time over the previous crew who came in with something more complex. Except if a crew came in with an 'alert' - something particularly serious like a cardiac arrest or serious trauma case where the hospital was fore warned of the crews arrival. In such cases, we all knew the lads would be some time before they cleared due to cleaning up the subsequent blood and snot that would adorn the walls of the ambulance.

Often, the second crew into hospital who cleared first would wait for the first to clear, and if sometimes they didn't, the second would reluctantly do so. There in started a phase of the first crews calling Metro control. Their transmission would consist of something such as,

"Metro control Raven 1......oh apologies, called in error".

The second crew, who could not hear the words of transmission from any other crews, only that a transmission had occurred, would hear Metro's reply with the caller's call sign. It would be presumed that the first crew sat next to them, had booked clear and were available for a job. They would then book themselves clear and available. And if there was only one job going, it would now automatically go to the second crew. Much to the amusement of the first who would hang out the windows and mock their colleagues. Another trick was to book clear as the first crew, but take the long route back to station if there were no other jobs at that time, thereby arriving back to station second and earning a place lower in the pile of boards for the next job instead of next out.

One evening, on the late shift of third manning, around 1989, I worked with Ted 'Chippy' Frankston from Henrietta Street, and his long standing crew mate Vince Manley. Also on their shift were Foxy and Bob. At some point in the shift we both ended up at Dudley Road Hospital, us having come in first. We both cleared around the same time, and Foxy and Bob waited for us to book up first. However, Chip had played an ace, by saying he'd just pop to the toilet first, instead going back into the casualty department, contacting Metro by phone, booking clear and actually getting a doctors urgent removal as our next case. This was the type of call which wasn't an emergency, but was more of a routine, non blue light case of picking up a patient from home, whose doctor had been out to them and subsequently arranged hospital admission. Chip returned to the truck, told Foxy we were on return to station, and subsequently started out. Our case was in the opposite direction to station and some distance out but believing us to be taking the long way home, and not being aware we had actually booked clear, they followed us in the hope of getting back to station after us and therefore being lower in the pack for getting the next job.

I could see them behind us laughing, obviously believing they had one up on us. But of course the laugh was ours. We drove and drove and drove, getting further and further from station, in fact around 20 miles from home and pulled up outside our designated address complete with second ambulance in tow. Suddenly realising they had been fooled as we got on the radio and booked in attendance at the job, which they could hear on their radio, they shot off at high speed, no doubt to try and get back somewhere near station before being discovered that they were so far away. The last laugh was ours. And the story had mileage for several days.

Not ending there though, three nights later, the same situation, with the same crews, arose by coincidence. This time, however, we didn't have a job, but instead told them at the hospital that we did. Foxy looked at Chip with suspicion, and clearly didn't know whether to believe him or not. They had been lucky the other day and hadn't been found out so far from home and didn't get into trouble. But clearly Foxy didn't want to push his luck again. We drove out of the hospital with them behind, clearly seeing where we would go.

With no job on the books and with it being 2 o'clock in the morning, we pulled up at a random house, where I'd been pre warned of the need to get out with the guys, approach the front door and knock on it. We duly pulled up outside 47 New Spring Street North, where I alighted the rear of the ambulance and with Vince and Chip leading, we walked up to the front door. Foxy and Bob had pulled up and were parked behind us with the engine running, and as the householder opened the front door rubbing his eyes, they drove off cursing us that we obviously had a job. I heard through the open door of our ambulance them booking clear and being told to return to station. Vince turned to the householder.

"Did you call for an ambulance mate?"

"Errrr...no...no, I don't think so," came the reply. He shouted up the stairs, "Carol, did you phone for an ambulance for your mother?"

A muffled reply said he had not, to which Vince replied that the hoax callers had obviously been at work again and that we were very sorry. We ran back to the ambulance and called clear so that Foxy and Bob would hear it. We could almost make out the names being called us from the other crew even though they were a mile or two nearer station than us. And upon return to station, although applauding the originality of the plot, they were still fuming. The last laugh was ours again. And this one had mileage for weeks! But we'd need to sleep with one eye open on nights, for revenge was always on the cards.

Riding supernumerary with the emergency crews was done on Friday or Saturday nights, whilst still working on the outpatient sector. I learned not to drop off to sleep when on these nights, as some of the horror stories I'd heard that the blokes had done to each other were horrendous, and something I felt being the newbie, I needed to be on my guard for. The more classic ones were done when people fell asleep, innocently removing their shoes before dozing off, only to invariably have them stolen, hidden and replaced with a large ladies size nine pink fluffy slipper, and the same size Wellington boot, clearly having been planned a few days before, for that particular individual so the size was right. They were bastards. You'd not see your shoes for the rest of the shift.

Another favourite if you kept your shoes on, was having your laces tied together when asleep, so when you jumped up in your slumber, you'd immediately fall flat on your face. Or the assailant would carefully pull down the fly zip of a blokes trousers, again while he was asleep, and pour warm water over his nether regions, then from the pay phone on station, call the red phone to which we had the number and was an ordinary outside line. The perpetrators would pretend to be asleep but would watch with slanted eyes the reaction when the guy got up, having checked his shoe laces were not tied first, and satisfied they were not, he would smugly walk across the mess room to answer the phone soon to become aware of the cooling wetness around his groin. It was usually not a small amount of water either. So if the receiver wasn't convinced he'd wet himself, he still had to go out of the station with a huge wet patch on the front of his trousers and undergo the subsequent embarrassment of trying to explain to the patient that he hadn't wet himself but that it was a prank played upon him. Health and safety issues never came into it, and neither was any real physical harm done, just a few pissed off blokes and a large amount of laughs.

Before my time, when Phil Oswald worked at Henrietta Street, his birthday was 'celebrated' by the blokes stripping him stark naked, and placing him into a Neil Robertson Stretcher. This was a rescue stretcher made from strips of wood lashed together with cloth tape to form a coffin shaped basket that the victim would be completely immobilised in and become totally unable to get out of themselves without help. It was used for rescuing the fallen from pits, holes and the like. However, on this occasion there was no injured faller. The naked Philip, facing backwards towards the oncoming traffic, was strapped, 'tackle out', onto the outside rear doors of an ambulance, which by the way was still on operational duty. The truck then drove around Birmingham city centre, for all to see. As if that wasn't bad enough, the guys then stopped outside a huge traffic island in the middle of town, took Phil off the rear doors but still in the stretcher, and propped him up against the doors of the central fire station, where, for the next half an hour, several hundred motorists were subjected to both Phil's where-for-all and his embarrassment. Eventually, the fire guys brought him back, where he continued his shift. And the favour to the fire guys would undoubtedly be returned soon, as this sort of behaviour was common place. Mopeds would be hoisted to the ceiling of the garage, and there was even an instance of a blokes car being put into a skip! Nothing was impossible with the right motivation, and evil set of thoughts. Needless to say, no one ever knew when my birthday was.

Stag do's were another time when, as the stag, your fate was sealed if the guests included an ambo. Being plastered, then being plastered up a lamp post! By that, I mean, being intoxicated, then following a trip to the local casualty department for some plaster of Paris and bandaging, meant the following morning, someone was going to wake up, hungover, having been plastered up a lamp post to the type with the protruding arm near the top. And a couple did, to be cut down, usually by the local fire service coming to the rescue yet again.

The men's toilets were often the scene of practical jokes set up by one of the blokes, Paul Bachelor. The 'traps' as they were known, or the individual toilet compartments would be locked, with the assailant climbing out over the door, so when Dave Peel, the boss, entered the gents for his morning ablutions, he would push open the main door, approach each trap, pushing it, mutter something under his breath then go out again thinking they were all in use. This would go on for a while until it was obvious someone was playing around. At which point you'd hear Dave's booming voice.

"BACHELOR YOU BASTARD!" Another favourite, was stretching cling film over the ladies individual toilets, before placing the seat down and getting out before one of the girls returned to station. And of course the first thing they'd do is run into the loo, stating loudly.

"Ooo gerout the way, I'm busting for a piss", as you'd hear them running up the corridor having run in from the garage. All the blokes, of course, would wait like giggly school boys for the scream. And sure enough, it would follow, to the howls of laughter from the mess room.

"BACHELOR, YOU BASTARD". His signature was always all over many of the pranks. Sitting on the bog became an anxious time, especially when you heard the creek of the door opening; water over the top of the trap doors, and lighted bangers underneath. His imagination knew few boundaries, and made for some very constipated blokes. I decided early in my career that it was best not to go at work. And definitely not if Bachelor was on.

CHAPTER 18.
POOR MEMORY.

Henrietta Street had a plethora of characters during my early days there. One such was Simon Johns. He was such a nice guy; the quiet type, who'd never hurt a fly, and always had cheery words and a smile for anyone and everyone he met. He'd never flare up if an obnoxious patient became abusive towards him, and I'm not even sure if he knew how. It just wasn't in his nature. He was at the opposite end of the spectrum of having a violent streak. He didn't take part in the issuing of blags, probably because he wasn't keen on receiving them, but did occasionally find himself on the receiving end. In many respects he was an ordinary bloke who turned up for duty, did his job to the best of his ability, then went home. But Simon was special; special because I doubt there is a person alive who is as laid back or as half soaked. He was famed for having the driving seat at an angle of about 50 degrees. How he could see the road and drive efficiently was, and still is a mystery to most of us that worked with him. But do it he did, and served his community to the tune of over 30 years.

One bitterly cold November night, Simon's rostered shift fell on nights, which were from 11pm to 7am. He duly turned up in his little car, and was telling the shift how long it had taken to defrost the windows due to the ice that was about in his neck of the woods. The conversation with the shift about defrosting windows went on for some time with various ideas being put into the pot.

"Why don't you leave the engine running for a while before you start out, and leave the heater running. Thats what I do, give it ten minutes and hey presto," said Simon's crew mate, Mick. Simon thought about the suggestion for a brief moment then replied.

"Ah well, I can't ya see, because my car's parked out on the grass verge outside my house, and you know what it's like round by me. If I left it running without me in it, it'd get nicked."

"Fair point," said Mick, "but you could do it while it's here at work in the morning. You know how the frost gets onto the cars when they're parked at the back of the station."

"Hmmm........ Yeah, good idea. I'll see what the windscreen is like in the morning".

So, that was that. A good simple plan, that can't go wrong. Right? Well, actually, where Simon was involved, it could, and did.

Upon return to station following a job at about half past six the following morning, as he drove past his car parked at the rear of the station, Simon noted the thick frost upon it as it had been a bitterly cold night with temperatures well sub zero. After parking the ambulance up in the garage, he went inside, fetched his car keys, and returned outside to his car where initially he had difficulties getting in because the locks were frozen. But after success, he started the engine and popped back inside the station for a final cuppa before finishing his shift and clocking out. But the combination of a warm drink, comfy chairs and tiredness at the end of his night shift, resulted in Simon dropping off to sleep. As was customary under these circumstances, particularly with Simon, as it happened on frequent occasions, at 7am, his shift mates all clocked out, leaving him still asleep. His mates usually had small wagers to see how long it would be before he woke up, his record being 10.30am.

On this occasion, at about 8 o'clock, he woke with a start, realised he'd 'overslept', put on his coat, walked out of the station front door, went across the road, and waited five minutes for the 67 bus, at which point he got on it. Outside his house he got off, did the short walk to his front door where his wife was about to walk the kids to school, before she then walked around the corner to work. He kissed them all, went inside and went to bed to sleep off his night shift, still completely oblivious.

Another of Simon's attributes was that the man could almost sleep upright, and would sleep well whenever he did. On this day he woke around four in the afternoon, pottered around the house, had tea and went to get ready for work. Thinking that he might have to spend some time defrosting the car again, he looked outside the bedroom window to check. And of course panicked when he didn't see the car. He dressed quickly and rushed downstairs opening the front door in case he'd been mistaken. But no, it still wasn't there. His wife, sensing his urgency came out side and they both looked up and down the road, but alas, it wasn't there. Stolen, obviously.

He got straight onto the police to inform them of the theft. Clearly the car had been taken from outside of the house, he stated, sometime between having arrived at home from work, and discovering the theft at about 8 pm. Simon decided that this was of such severity that he couldn't possibly come in to work that evening, so phoned the station and spoke to Jackie Stow, the leading hand. The conversation went something like this;

"Oh, hello, Jack, it's Simon here. Listen, I've got some trouble, my car's been stolen and I've got to go down to the police station and all, so I won't be in for my night shift."

There was a brief silence before Simon could hear Jack's

wheezing giggle.

"I was wondering when you'd phone. You've done it again, and this time it's a corker. Yer bloody car is still parked out the back of the station where you left it this morning. It's been ticking over all day. They'll be no bloody petrol left in it!"

Simon had the embarrassment of contacting the police to tell them of the mistake, and had to apologise for the inconvenience his poor memory had caused. Not to mention the fact that his cars' registration number was being sought by half of the Birmingham traffic police.

CHAPTER 19. A LEGGE UP TO BLOOD, GUTS AND GORE.

The initial 6 week training course to get onto front line was followed by a steady period of development. Initial cases I attended were a hazy mix of confusion, trial and error, where the experienced guys would 'point me in the right direction'. This ranged from a subtle handing me the oxygen equipment where I'd delayed or forgotten to administer, right through to an out and out bollocking, usually for something minor, but often in front of the patient and their relatives. I of course felt bloody awful and very embarrassed in these circumstances but this wasn't often and these occasions became less and less as my abilities grew. My mentors in these few occasions were often bully types and knew I would accept my fate from them. These were the still the days of a militaristic service where the gaffers were referred to as 'sir', and some would turn up to work with their boots so bulled shiny, you could have shaved in them.

My first year development consisted of three months on the road, followed by a weeks 'in-service' with a training officer to assess my progress. I would be crewed up with another trainee, and we would work on front line in the usual manner but be over seen by a trainer who would start out watching us like a hawk, and then once confident in our progress and abilities, would relax back and let us get on with things. There'd be an occasional question popped through from their perch in the back of the ambulance

"So tell me about diabetes then." Or "how would you treat someone having a fit?" We'd take it in turns to answer over the week and as the trainers were all good blokes, we found it useful.

On my second period of in-service training, I was crewed up with Alan Collins, a round faced bloke of my age who I'd started with some three years earlier. His cheeks were always rosy with a wispy mop of dark curly hair adorning the top of his head and his voice had a vague Irish tint gained from his birth place. He was always jolly and we laughed a great deal. I really enjoyed working with him.

Our in service training officer for the week was Frank Legge. Frank was a serious bloke on the outside but with a gentle inner, and who was definitely on the side of the student. A clean shaven bloke with a slight Scottish accent and impeccable dress. Every morning of the week, we'd all meet up at Henrietta Street Ambulance Station where the training vehicle would be waiting for us, and a coffee later we'd be serving the public of Birmingham and sorting their crises and problems, hopefully in an efficient and compassionate manner.

One midmorning found us having dropped off a patient at The General Hospital. We were parked up in the bay, chatting through the case we'd just completed.

"So," Frank broke the short silence with, "Bradders how do you think that went?" I turned my mouth down, and my gaze up as I continued.
"Ok……..I think." Then as now, I hated having to publicly state my performance as being acceptable, however this was the arena. To temper my conscience, my brain went into overdrive for elements of the job which hadn't gone so well. "But I should

have asked more about his condition. Why is it that we always ponder on stuff after the job that we should have done or asked?" Frank came back.

"Well lad, thats the duty of experience. It'll come. You're young yet. But remember, you should always look back on all your jobs and realise that there was something, however small, you could've done better for your patient." Wise words indeed and a property I would both remember for myself and my students in years to come.

Our conversation was cut short when a Henrietta Street crew who been in the hospital after us for a brief time, then drove passed us and stopped. Out jumped one of the guys and approached Frank in our driving seat. its

"Seeing as you blokes are on training, you might wanna follow us to the mortuary. Got one you might find interesting" he said. The mortuary was just across the road from the General Hospital and served to house, as the name suggests, the deceased of the area. Protocol at the time instructed us to transport most of our deceased patients who died either at home or who'd met their demise in a public place to this mortuary. My adrenaline spiked wondering what was interesting about this case, and without knowing what were about to experience or the cause of their death, we duly followed the other ambulance the 200 yards to The Birmingham City Mortuary.

They'd arrived just a few seconds or so before us and were both already out of the front seats and opening the back doors of their truck. We pulled up behind them. Now looking directly into the rear saloon, all I could see were about six bags, each the size of black bin liners and in the lack of light they all looked quite dark. I was puzzled. Whey the hell were these blokes moving rubbish bags to the mortuary? Was it another prank?

Once inside the building, with the light now so much better, all became horribly clear. The bags were clear, thick polythene. Some were rounded and full, others only partly filled and with odd shaped contents. One of the blokes broke the silence.

"Redcliffe Station. Jumped in front of an express train." He didn't need to say anymore. It all became disgustingly obvious. Up to this point, my experience of death and destruction had been limited, but hadn't included anything of such traumatic explosion. Sat in front of me was a human corpse, in six plastic bags, and anatomically unrecognisable from across the room. The statutory exclamation of "urgghhhh" emanated from both Alan and myself and we were herded nearer the bags to get a better view by Frank. Muscle, bone, clothing, hair, blood, bowel and snot were presented before us. My excitement turned to slight nausea. Here was I, fresh-faced and who only a few years before had still been in school, was now in the thick of sights and experiences that humans shouldn't really be dealing with. Trying to give an air of not being affected by this, I cautiously stepped closer to the bags. One of them took my eye in particular. It had something inside which initially looked recognisable, but I wasn't sure. I got right up to the bag and poked it with my finger in an investigative manner, turning my head to the side. I still couldn't fathom which part of this poor bugger I was looking at. I poked again, this time a little more firmly. The piece of flesh I was studying then turned slightly and fell towards me so it was right up against the inside of the bag. I stepped back slightly, now with fear and the reality that I was looking at half of a male face. Part of an ear, an upper lip adorned with a wisp of moustache hair, cheek tissue, part of a jaw with teeth and an eye. The eye. This was all of a sudden what gave this sight an emotive feel. The eye gave him identification as once a person. It starred at me like some weird cyclops monster, the jaw so displaced from the eye that it almost resembled a smile. This sudden exposure made me take a rather quick step backwards in a mixture of disbelief and fright. Never had I had such a baptism of fire and been exposed to such gore. It would be the first of many though I'm afraid.

This post mortal experience had left Alan and I in a rather sombre mood; I think both of us questioned our decision to join up, knowing this would be the first of many. Frank however, remained his usual cheery self, and suggested we consider where to eat lunch, which I found bizarre. How could he be so obtuse? Of course, it wasn't until I became more experienced that I really understood this. I know many of my students have actually been through the same with me since, and we've discussed it. It's at times like these that experience has taught me not to get involved in the emotions of the event; who was he? Did he have family? Did he step out in front of the train by accident or was it suicide? These kind of questions provoke too much thought; the kind of thought that fills the stress bucket. The kind of thought that has this experience come back to haunt you either straight after or in 20 years. See it visually for what it is, take an anatomical lesson from it and move on. Don't get emotionally involved.

Later that day we were due to finish shift at 3pm. Alan had been telling us earlier about an appointment he had late afternoon and didn't want to miss. So when Metro Control gave us a 999 job at ten minutes to 3pm from the station, Alan stayed and Frank and myself covered it.

We were called to a tower block in Highgate, to a report of a female patient having abdominal pains. Frank drove and within five minutes we were pulling up outside the block. At the time, the vehicles we used were the 'traditional' types; painted white with a red stripe down each side and twin stretchers, one down each side, with double opening rear doors. Equipment carried was sparse by modern standards.

We alighted the vehicle and with some excitement, I looked at the tower block. A reminder of twenty years before when these establishments provided modern housing for the working class away from the back to back slums. These had their own bathrooms and heating. Walls of windows and concrete of plain grey, with the occasional colour on the balconies of drying washing to break up the drab sight. A lone barking dog way up on one of the higher floors signified the type of housing this represented; an inner city and lower socio-economic life style.

A few steps from the ambulance saw us standing before the wooden entrance doors. The security locks were long since broken off and people walked in and out at will. Clearly anybody could enter, and many did who didn't live there to supply the varied activities that went on in the block; drugs and prostitution mainly but only in a few of the flats. Most were good law abiding people who lived amongst these few individuals who would bring the whole place down. Opening of the entrance doors revealed a certain smell that seems particular to these tower blocks. It's a mixture of Jeyes fluid, filth, faeces, urine and body odour, but in fairness is tolerable once you get used to it, and always remains the same, no matter what tower block you find yourself in. Inside the door, a shopping trolley lay on its side and we had to negotiate around it to approach the lift.

I went to press the lift button. Frank interjected.

"Don't forget Bradders, don't press the button with your finger, only the end of your pen."

"Yep, got that one Frank," as I pressed the button with my pen. There had been a notice come round the stations warning both ambulance and midwife staff that there had been occasions where lift buttons and handrails had been discovered to have used drug needles bent into 'u' shapes and glued into them using chewing gum and that there had been instances of needle stick injuries as a result. Consequently, ambos and nurses now pressed these buttons with a pen, not a finger.

We waited patiently in front of the lift door, while a clattering and clanking from the lift shaft above us signalled it getting ever nearer to the ground floor. The unnerving noise got louder until the lift arrived whereupon this decrepit box stopped, and for several seconds nothing happened. No doors opened leaving me wondering what was going on. Then with another loud scraping sound, the doors slowly opened, to reveal another semi-repulsive odour. We stepped in. I'd kind of gotten used to this kind of environment, having worked these tower blocks now for several months. This particular one was actually relatively clean; although no mop had traversed the floor for several millennia. There was a distinct lack of dirty nappies, pools of urine and the odd human turd adorning the corner. However, this still didn't appease my concern of whether this lift would actually get us to the chosen floor.

Our destination was flat number 47, but what we didn't know was, which floor this was situated on. No markings inside the lift left us wondering, so as a guess I pressed the sixth floor button with the end of my pen. I reminded myself not to ever henceforth suck the aforementioned writing implement for fear of contracting something deadly. The doors trundled to a close, then again nothing for what appeared an age before it started ascending. The same, but now louder scraping noises ensued for floor after floor until we reached the sixth. The stop was superseded again by the statutory unwillingness to open. The kind of delay that sets claustrophobia off, wondering if I should have told the kids I loved them before I left for work this morning.

Luck was on our side. This was the floor we needed, and I held a slight smugness knowing that my knowledge of traversing these inner city tower blocks was improving with time. This 'guess the floor the flat is on' would prove to be invaluable in the years to come. Frank's approach remained the same throughout all this; remaining still and maintaining his stare forward. He refused to look down in the lift, refused to alter his facial expression, and never appeared to sniff the aroma. I reckoned his coping mechanism was to imagine he was in the lift of Harrods or some millionaires condominium, where one could get a shoe shine or a cocktail while in the lift.

We'd already decided that this job was mine, so I approached the front door of number 47, a heavy wooden affair, with the remnants of a door bell and one number missing but the outline still clearly visible. While Frank stood behind me, I rattled the letterbox and stood there with confidence. Deep within the flat I could hear footsteps walking slowly down the hallway until they were right behind the door. Keys turned, latches were disengaged, and bolts were slid in a Fort Knox type way, such was the environment of inner city tower blocks of the era in Birmingham. The door slowly opened to little more than ajar with a chain remaining in situ, and a young woman's face appeared and moved from side to side in the slim opening, scanning us with suspicion. I broke the silence.

"Hello, it's the ambulance." I waited for a response, but the staring and moving from side to side continued for a few more seconds. The door closed, and the chain was slid off of its holding and the door cautiously re-opened. In front of us stood a very thin, young woman, I guessed around mid 20's, with straight, greasy and unwashed dark hair. She wore no makeup and had a distinct look of fear on her face.

"I'm ……errr…..bleeding," she said quietly with hesitation. She looked back into the flat with a fear about her before turning back around to face me. It was obvious that she meant that her bleeding was vaginal. I continued.

"Ok, well what's your name? I'm Dave and this is Frank, pointing over my shoulder.

"Please be quiet and speak in a whisper," she came back. "Or he might wake," turning her head to the left to point towards the inner sanctum of the flat. Even in my inexperience, it was clear to me that she was in an abusive relationship and her demeanour implied the other half was inside the flat and was not aware she'd phoned for the ambulance, and was presumably asleep.

A closer look at the woman revealed she'd been crying and a red mark high on her cheek looked like it had been caused by a punch. I asked again.

"What's your name?"

"Please don't tell him I called you, will you?" She replied, not really listening to me but clearly absolutely petrified of some monster within the flat. I sensed I needed to be both compassionate and understanding but assertive with this poor lady, and clearly her door step was not the place to remain. There are times when as ambulance staff, we stay on scene for extended periods of time, and occasions when we move the patient rapidly and the latter was going to get her away from this environment that was making her uneasy. That would make managing her far more effective.

"Come on," I said. "Let's pop you down to the hospital." And she followed us out into the communal hallway, quietly closing her front door, and to where the lift was still waiting as the doors once again noisily opened.

In the relative safety of the lift, she seemed to snap out of the total fear state she'd displayed a few minutes earlier and woke up.

"My name's Cindy."

"Well Cindy we're going to get you sorted and pop you down to the hospital," I replied."How long have you been bleeding?"

"A couple of hours," she said still not looking me in eye, preferring to gaze down at the floor. I continued.

"And how much blood are you loosing? Are we talking about the same as a period?"

"Urrrm, well I've had to use several pads already, and this one feels like it's quite wet." The lift clanged to a halt on the ground floor and after a few seconds the door opened with a loud scraping noise.

Frank opened the rear doors of the ambulance and Cindy was directed to sit on the side facing stretcher as was customary at the time. Frank quickly closed the doors and walked with purpose to the drivers seat. We were well over our finishing time and I sensed he wanted to go home. The drive would only be a short one of five minutes to the General Hospital and more questions ensued from me to Cindy. It turns out she'd discovered she was pregnant, and had told her boyfriend earlier in the day. He became angry and an argument ensued where upon he repeatedly punched and kicked her in the abdomen, then started drinking and had fallen asleep. Cindy subsequently developed pain and bleeding.

It was during this questioning with her that I noticed blood dripping from the underside of her upper leg and dropping onto the floor. Cindy seemed oblivious to this and carried on talking and I didn't want to alert her to the fact and cause more grief. But the bleeding was worsening and within minutes was now almost a stream. In my total inexperience, I didn't know what to do aside of stick my head through to Frank in the front and let him quietly know. We were only yards from the hospital and so continued, but by now there appeared so much blood the pool was moving up and down, and side to side in the saloon with every brake and turn, and Frank, sensing this was serious clearly started driving faster. Another look at Cindy's leg and this bleeding was now a constant stream. I re-informed Frank, seeking guidance but his concentration was getting the patient to hospital, and upon arrival, a wheelchair was duly sought along with a word in the ear of the receiving nursing sister who quickly made provision for Cindy to be taken into the resuscitation room within the casualty department.

With the patient delivered, there was some clearing up to do. The floor of the ambulance looked like we'd had an amputated leg from a hit and run, such was the amount of blood which by now was coagulating. Frank had an air of impatience at the time I was taking to clean up and very soon we were back on the road driving to Henrietta Street to clock off. Nothing was said on the way back and in my inexperience I didn't ask any questions. I was keen to know however if I could have done more. I'd felt totally helpless and wanted to learn what to do for the next time I would come across such obstetric bleeding. In hindsight, and with the benefit of better understanding now, there were few elements of the case that went well.

Rapidly leaving the scene was a good thing, although I realise now it was less to do with the patient and more to allow Frank to go home. But the patient should not have been allowed to walk, and should have been laid down on the stretcher perhaps with feet raised. Pain relief should have been offered, and without doubt, Frank, as a qualified paramedic should have taken control of my ineptitude. In fairness, obstetric bleeding cannot be compressed and the provision of intravenous fluids was less beneficial to the patient than getting her to the definitive place of care - the hospital, and quickly. But this was also the time period where Frank's paramedicine was still in its infancy.

This job highlighted to me the importance of forgetting one's own circumstances and issues, to concentrate on the patients condition, and provide the care that should have been given. A crew fucks up as a crew. Her condition may have been worsened by her management, and Frank should have known better. He was both experienced and a training officer to a green student who didn't know any better. These were the days before any fancy treatments that we now give, but her condition required simple positioning and a bit of common sense. It was a learning curve for me, and carried lessons and principles that remain with me to this day. Many a clinician has lost their job trying to cut corners to go home 15 minutes earlier. However, I've never heard of anyone being criticised for over treating or doing the job properly. My guide since Cindy has always been that if I stand in front of the Coroner following a patient of mine who died, can I justify what I did or did not do? The answer must always be yes. Even if it means finishing late, performing some time consuming procedure or going outside of the rule book.

In Cindy's case, she went to theatre and was fixed with no lasting issue. I went to the same address a year or so later for a male and she was there. I didn't feel like she recognised me but it seemed strange that she was still within this same abusive relationship. With little understanding of the psychology of these toxic environments, I attended a lady some time later in another tower block where the doors and walls had holes in them, and who had the results of having been assaulted by her partner with the statutory black eye and cut lip. She asked if her partner could come with her and he seemed calm enough to be allowed to do so, particularly as she claimed she'd 'walked into a door by accident'. En route to hospital, sat next to him, she admitted that he'd punched her, just like he does frequently. He had a slightly embarrassed look on his face as she chastised him about it. But shortly after arrival at hospital the pair of them walked out, hand in hand before she'd been seen, and back into the arms of the abuser.

It was to be many years later that I would gain at least some understanding of why the abused often stays with the abuser. Threats of more violence, promises that it won't happen again and just because the abused loves the abuser and 'they can't help it' or 'they're stressed', or its the abused's fault, for saying the wrong thing. Narcissism, control and personality however, are often the real reasons why they abuse.

CHAPTER 20.
ONE UNDER.

In 1990, the gaffer of Henrietta Street, was Dave Peel. He was a big, tall, thick set man with a stand-up comic sense of humour, that became his hallmark. In all the years I knew Dave, he always cracked a joke, or did something funny every time I spoke to him, in some shape or form. Always very fair, I liked him a lot, and my respect for him knew no boundaries.

When I first started in the ambulance service, I received much contempt from many of the front line guys just for being on outpatients and obviously not worthy of being in their presence. Dave, at this time, was a leading hand at Sutton Coldfield. He offered me compassion, friendship, guidance and always a smiling face. He mentored and advised me, and was the first person to show me how to make up a stretcher, getting me to do it again and again until I got it right. He instilled into me that the back of my ambulance, no matter whether it was an emergency or non emergency one, gave off an impression that would kill or cure my patient. If the sick saw a scruffy stretcher they'd lose confidence in my abilities. But if they were to see a smart, well made and clean bed in the rear of a smart clean ambulance, then their confidence would be elevated and would allow me to get away with elements I didn't know and would potentially be winging. This principle was in turn passed on by me to hundreds of students during my time as a tutor, and in deed remains with me today, as I continue to instil it to student paramedics I come across. My stretcher and vehicle still looks good today and would be fit for a prince to be cared for in, all thanks to Dave. My respect for this man continues today. He retired in 2012 having worked into his fourth decade for the ambulance service. With him went the character, the person, the humour, and although now living on the opposite side of the world from him, we still keep in touch. On a visit to the UK at Christmas 2012, I popped in to see him as I always do, and we found ourselves reminiscing and laughing about characters in the bygone era.

At the time Dave was the boss at Henrietta Street, I'd completed my front line training and was now working on the emergency ambulances. One morning on a day shift I was crewed up with Ted Frankston, but known as Chip. We both arrived for work at the back of the station, parking our cars in their usual places and walking up the back steps into the station. It was clear to me from seeing Chip, that something wasn't quite right with him. He seemed slightly uneasy and every so many paces, his legs changed their normal walking position with his right knee elevating higher than usual for that step. I was still the new boy, and Chip the old hand, so it wasn't my place to be asking him if everything was ok. But that aside, he seemed pretty much normal so I didn't give it any more thought. Chip was another of the big men; sporting a crew cut and with a tough look, he was as hard as a coffin nail and nothing phased him. He was a black belt in karate, and wasn't one you'd want to pick a fight with, having the stereo typical bouncer look that you'd not want to get on the wrong side of. I often imagined him wearing a long black overcoat standing behind Vinnie Jones, or appearing on the set of films like 'Lock Stock and 2 Smoking Barrels' or 'love, Honour and Obey', as a gang style minder. Chip had actually done some bouncing in his time and was apparently pretty good at it. But despite his appearance, he was a true gentleman and quite old fashioned in his mannerisms. He'd always hold the door for a lady, or give up his seat for someone elderly or infirm. I guess you'd call him a big softy at heart.

This particular morning was quiet for us, and after a cursory vehicle check I settled down into the empty mess room for some breakfast, when Dave, the boss, came in for his. Ted got out of his seat, and was clearly in some discomfort as he walked across the room, heading for the kitchen.

"You alright Ted?", Dave said with some concern.

"No I'm not". Chip's reply came with a hint of severity, his voice low and booming."But don't ask!"

With the corner of a bacon sandwich poised to be shoved into his mouth, Dave turned his head and looked at me. He leaned a little in my direction, raised his eyebrows and with an impish grin developing he spoke in a hushed tone.

"Must be his ceramics on the move again."

In my naivety, I didn't know what this meant, so in the same hushed tone, as I had at least guessed that whatever it did mean, it wasn't going to be complimentary to Chip, I asked.

"Ceramics?"

Now with a mouthful of butty, Dave continued.

"Ceramic tiles. Piles. Obviously playing him up again."

At this I tried to stifle my laughter, and I was doing alright until Dave spoke up again. Ted was by now walking with almost a limp, and every other step was still raising his right knee quite high. He looked like he was trying to impersonate Max Wall, and by now had his hand down his trousers, frantically doing something with his 'tackle'.

"Ted, if the crabs are giving you grief again, I've got some cream that'll help."

Ted's tone moved slightly towards that of humour, allowing

me to laugh louder and of which I was grateful. He started to grin as he looked at Dave and I.

"And you two can shut the fuck up. You've no idea of the discomfort I'm goin through"

"So what you done then", continued Dave as he tried to wipe some ketchup from his tie that had shot out of his sandwich.

"Never you bloody mind, ya pair of fuckers. But it's bloody uncomfortable" retorted Ted, who by now was heading out of the mess room. He turned left towards the toilets chuntering to himself. "I've had enough of this......."

Dave and I finished our breakfast with a quietening chuckle over Ted's misfortune. Whatever had been the cause of it, we were about to graced with. Ted's footsteps on the wooden floor as he walked down the corridor towards the gents, had sounded like the hunchback of Notre Dame, scraping his right leg and hopping every other step on his left. But a few minutes later, we heard normal, steady footprints returning back up the corridor and seconds later, Teds beaming face came into view round the door frame in the kitchen as I looked through the serving hatch from the mess room. No limp, and no raised right leg with every other step. Whatever had been troubling him, clearly wasn't now. Ted popped some bread under the grill.

"I tell ya, that's better", he said with some clear relief on his face. My curiosity was building, but I was beaten to asking by Dave.

"Ted, what the bloody 'ell was wrong? You come into work, looking like you've been starring in the Ministry of Funny Walks pantomime, leavin' me and the boy thinking you got anything from piles to pubic lice".

Ted approached the serving hatch, looked directly at us, and in a quiet voice started speaking.

"If this gets out, I'll know where it's come from........but.......when I got up this mornin it was dark, and the wife, she'd 'ad a late night last night so I didn't want to put the light on to get dressed. Well......I opened the draw where me underpants are kept, and took out what I thought was a pair of them new pants that Mary had bought me for Christmas. I thought they was a bit small and tight but I put 'em on anyway, and when I just been into the shit 'ouse to check, I had a pair of Mary's skimpy knickers on."

At this me and Dave burst out laughing. What made it funnier was the image of this big, hard, no nonsense bloke wearing a pair of ladies knickers!

Dave piped up after the laughter started to subside.

"Yeah don't worry Ted, no one will know. It'll be our little secret"

"Ya couple of fuckers" now also laughing and definitely seeing the funny side of things, "I'm not going to hear the end of this am I?" And he didn't. Twenty some odd years later, the story is still being told......

Chip and myself had just finished a job at the hospital when we booked clear. It was a cold autumn morning and the skies were grey and the air damp. I was looking forward to the drive back to station where I knew a cuppa would await to warm us up. But fate had something other than a cup of tea in mind.

"Metro control Eagle 4?" Our radio startled out following a short period of silence. "Got a treble nine for you at the Hospital railway station. Not sure what's going on there but there's some kind of incident".

It wasn't unusual to get limited information about the details of a 999 call at that time, and we often then, as now, find ourselves going into situations with little or no knowledge of what we are about to face. But this was one case I was not prepared for. I was still a novice, having only been out of training school for some six months. My experience was growing but I had a long way to go, and I often think now, that as a paramedic, there is always something I haven't seen, always something I haven't dealt with, and always something I haven't experienced. My career is therefore one of a journey, not a destination. And here, in 1990, I was a very young 24 year old working in a very bad, grown up world, where people hurt each other and children and adults die. No one should have to see and bear witness to the sights and experiences that ambulance staff are exposed to. But they do.

We made our way the mile or so to the train station. I remember Chip saying something about bloody train commuters fainting on the platform. Apparently he'd had a run of them in the previous few months, most of whom had recovered before he'd arrived so he felt he'd had a wasted journey. One of the things this job taught me was never to assume. Remember that saying of mine that 'assumption is the mother of all fuck ups'? Well it was here too. Running through my mind was a young lady, sat on a chair on the platform recovering well from her faint, with the station ticket man telling us he'd phoned the lady's husband and he was going to come and collect her, so we could return to station for that cuppa I'd set my heart on. In a cocky way, I'd sort of shut off a little; a very dangerous thing to do as a front line ambulance man, and something which we all have to constantly be on our guard for.

We pulled up outside of the station, and as Chip applied the click click click of the handbrake and the engine died, I became horribly aware of an eery silence unusual for this particular station. You might almost say it was deafening. I've come across this silence dozens of times since and now know it to mean only one thing; death. But not ordinary death, but man verses big machine death. Mutilation death of the vilest kind.

On this job, I was attending, and as my colleague jumped out of the drivers side, I slid my door open, to be met by a bloke in a British Rail uniform wearing a look of horror and panic on his face.

"Come quickly", he said, "I don't know if the poor buggers still alive".

My heart went into over drive, but still I didn't know what the situation was. Chip, as cool as a cucumber, leaned over towards and across me and spoke to the bloke,

"Is it one under mate?" To which the confirmation came. Chip looked at me, and in a very nonchalant way said,

"Well, just like delivering a baby, we all have a first time. It's gonna be messy so prepare yourself."

I grabbed the oxygen box and first aid bag, and followed the guy past a crowd of people and down the ramp towards the track. Chip confirmed with him that all the trains had been stopped and the power had been turned off. Reminiscing the case, I remember thinking that I'd done the session in training school on rail incidents and what the priorities are at them, but at the time completely forgot what they were. I was in 'headless chicken' mode and it was only for the experience and calm handling from Chip that kept me safe. At the platform there was a stationary commuter train with about three or four carriages. It had stopped short of where it should be, so the end carriages were hanging off the far end of the platform, where a couple of police officers and another British Rail man stood looking at us, and on the platform opposite there was no one. silence abounded and you could have heard a pin drop. I gained the impression that the two of us were centre stage, that all eyes were on us, and the sight of those people I could see standing with their hands in their pockets didn't bode well. If my patient had have been obviously alive, I would have expected to have seen these people busy, doing something, running around and calling to us to hurry up. But they weren't.

We were led to the engine end of the platform where a small ladder led off the concrete to allow access down onto the track. Chip stood behind me and made no effort for the ladder. I gleaned the impression this one was my job, my inception; my baptism of blood. Maybe, like hunting my first fox, with the hounds, I'd get my forehead 'blooded'. I was centre stage and there was no getting out. Not that I wanted to, but then again, with a wave of nausea over me, perhaps I did.

This one was real; very real. There was a point in this stage of my career where attending these sort of cases produced fear and nausea, which instantly disappeared when I started being busy. but at this point I wasn't busy, and there was nothing to occupy me to take away this feeling of impending and rising vomit. I forced myself forward, reluctantly, with every step. I negotiated the ladder, walking backwards for the half dozen rungs until I could hear the crunch of the oily gravel under foot.

"Round the other side" shouted the railman, "over there."

I looked up at him then turned my head in the direction of his finger to the far side of the carriages from the platform, and what appeared to be the second or third carriage. Trying to appear experienced and unfazed by what I thought I was going to see, I gathered my composure and walked around the front of the engine, with Chip close on my heels. I reckoned he was close enough to catch me if I'd fainted. And maybe that was why he was so close. But as I rounded the engine to look down the line of the train I was surprised to see nothing. I'd expected to see a pair of legs sticking out from under the wheels of the train, and experienced a very short lived euphoria, as if this had all been a big joke and there was to be no blood, guts and gore. But as my gaze worked back along the train, I spotted something blue near a wheel about 30 feet away from me. I walked towards it, and finally standing level with this blue thing, I realised very quickly what I was looking at.

It was a coat wrapped tightly around one of the train wheels. Along with it was a mass of hair, flesh, clothing, blood and muscle, all mixed up so I couldn't determine which bit was what. Instead of the fear, puke and revulsion I was expecting, I'd hit the 'busy' stage, and found it fascinating, drawing me in closer. I could see an arm, twisted, broken and emerging over one of the tracks, with silvery, shiny bone protruding and congealing blood hanging from it in the silence. Looking further under the train and towards its rear, was a leg, severed above the knee, and exposing stringy sinew, more shiny bone and bits of flesh. Light pink coloured blobs of what looked like fish roe was splattered over the wooden sleepers. This was the same as I'd seen with my 'jumper' weeks earlier, and I knew to be brain tissue. Every so many feet, sections of skull, with hair still attached littered the oil soaked stones between the sleepers. There was no doubt as to the fate of this person. But man or woman, I couldn't tell. My oxygen and first aid bag wouldn't be needed here. And as riveted as I was at this scene, I was glad I didn't have to help get the body out from under there. Cases of death like this are treated as a crime scene until otherwise proven, and are dealt with by the police and coroners office, so our job with this person was complete.

Having seen the results of train verses person at the mortuary, in the six plastic bags some months before, that seemed like an anatomy and physiology lesson. There was no emotion, no scene to picture. Just body parts. That days case was so very different. Here there was an environment, people, smells, comments and emotion. Here I could have an imagination as to what it must have looked and felt like when this poor individual stepped off the platform. What did it sound like at point of impact? Did the body explode? It all seemed surreal.

We were asked to have a look at the train driver who not surprisingly, was quite shocked by the incident. Sat on a chair in the station waiting room well away from the train, he appeared physically uninjured, but had a visible tremor and struggled to hold a mug of tea still that someone had given him, so the contents slopped and splashed onto the floor. But he didn't want to go to hospital. Alarmingly, he described how, as he was pulling into the station, a young man stood on the edge of the platform, and at the last minute, looked him straight in the eye and jumped in front of the train, so he'd had no chance of pulling up before the man fell under the wheels. Later, pondering on the job, I thought it one thing to commit suicide but another to involve some innocent bystander with such emotion as this poor guy was suffering. The train driver would see this man starring into his eyes for a long time to come.

Some years later, purely by coincidence, and as so often happens, I came across another attempted suicide by deliberate overdose of tablets. These cases amounted to several a week sometimes, and although they all received the same compassion, they were a regular occurrence and could get monotonous. As part of gaining an accurate clinical history and the development of a rapport with the patient, I would try to ascertain what they had done in their attempt to kill themselves and why they wanted to do it. Often they wouldn't speak and we'd end up merely providing some comfort and transport. Many times though, it was the proverbial cry for help, and I got pretty good at determining if I was dealing with a genuine failed attempt, an attention seeker or a lost soul in need of real help and support.

On this occasion the guy informed me that he had made a couple of previous attempts at suicide because he was chronically depressed and could see no way out. He hadn't worked in seven years following an incident at work. Apparently, he'd been a train driver who'd been haunted by killing someone who'd stared into his eyes before jumping off the platform at Hospital rail station some years before........

CHAPTER 21.
JUMPERS

The early days of my career saw some horrendous trauma. This was brought about largely because vehicle technology hadn't advanced to the level it is today. Remember this was over 35 years ago. Cars crashing in 1988 were designed and built in the 60's and 70's; no airbags, no crumple zones, and a seat belt law that was only enforced in the UK two years earlier, and was barely adhered to by many vehicle occupants. Cars such as Escorts, Minis, Marinas and Maxis saw people trapped by engines and dashboards heading rear wards in head on collisions, and rear seat passengers 'submarining' under the front seats, ending up in such unnatural positions that survival was hopeless. These vehicles were designed with what seemed no thought for occupant survival, and I make no apology for describing such atrocities. Today vehicle design is so much better. Airbags, engines that submarine under the car instead of coming backwards into the compartment, side impact protection systems, roll over protection systems and mobile phones that detect accidents and automatically call the emergency services. It's been many years since I've asked the Fire Service to perform a dash roll, a half roof removal or ram a door pillar.

Another type of call we used to see a lot of too during these times was the jumper. Poor individuals whose lives had reached such a low that they sought to commit suicide by jumping off buildings. Birmingham then, unlike now was littered with high rise tower blocks built largely in the 60's to combat the housing slums of the turn of the 20th century which now could provide for the needs of the people to provide them with quality housing. As I've already eluded to, these blocks became a living nightmare for many. Crammed into small spaces and a breeding ground for drugs, prostitution and at the very least noisy neighbours. They were a low socio-economic level. Hardly surprising then that mental health in some stooped to the level of suicide from various causes and not made any better by their living conditions.

There were certain tower blocks which seemed to have been more prevalent for jumpers than others. One such block sited near the old Accident Hospital in Birmingham, known as 'The Accy', was the site of many a drama of this type. There were instances of crews being called to a jumper, horrendously injured from this block who would be transported across the road to the Accy, only to get another jumper from the same tower block some thirty minutes later.

In 1988 The West Midlands Ambulance Service employed a few 'fast track' individuals to fill a growing need for front line staff. I'd joined a year earlier, desperate to get into the elitism of emergency work, but had to serve my time on the out patient, 'granny runs'. So these few that were taken on who bypassed me and several of my colleagues were viewed with disparity and dislike. From a personal perspective, I had way less of an issue with the individuals and more with the service, where I couldn't fathom why some idiot would think that it was a good idea to take someone off the street, and push them through a pathway with less foundation and knowledge, rather than promote from within. A few out patient staff were never destined to make the grade but many of us were.
One such individual was Johnny. All of us on out patients took an immediate dislike to him, but largely this was due to his pathway rather than the person. The Union created a

stink and poisoned us against him. He'd clearly come from an educated background and was actually a nice bloke, and once the novelty had worn off, I rather liked him. He was quite posh and had an air of upper class about him, but he didn't class himself as such. He was confident and a good communicator and being of a similar age to myself we got on well once the ice had been broken. I found myself on my six week front line training course not too long after Jon and although I was allocated to C shift, of which he wasn't, we did find ourselves working together from time to time.

April 1990 saw me starting work on an early shift with him. Spring was a little late and the mornings were still a little crisp and chilly, more so for me as I commuted to work in those days by motorbike. Having removed my bike gear I headed for the mess room, where a bacon sandwich and a steaming cup of tea would be waiting for me, made by Ken, the station hand who did everything from cooking to cleaning and was loved by all. Jon was already in and looked as keen as mustard, as we greeted each other. He was my senior in terms of experience as he'd been on for nearly a year, to my few months and although I was still green behind the ear, Jon was advancing well and I felt confident we could handle most things that might me thrown at us that day.

We were a few motors back for a job in a mess room of staff as the morning started quietly, and the chink of snooker balls broke the air from time to time, the television blurred in the background and the hazy smell of pipe smoke carried above the table where I was seated. Each time the phone rang with a job, my heart would race and I'd look up in excitement wondering what the crew were going out to. The older blokes would talk down the phone, some polite, others not so, with an occasional "uh huh" or "right", then put the phone down and saunter out to the garage where I'd hear their vehicle start up and meander out. The blue beacons spinning on the roof as I looked out of the mess room window would fire my jealousy of what they'd be going to, then a minute or so later the familiar sound of the two tone air horns would signify they'd reached the traffic lights at Snow Hill.

Roles of attending or driving were switched half way through the shift. On this particular morning Jon and I had been allocated 'The Beast'. Remember the race I'd been involved in some while earlier before I moved up on to front line? A V8 engined Freight Rover monster that in comparison with the older Fords, was quicker. But it came at a price. Handling was terrible, with very soft suspension and these trucks had a tendency to roll badly in the corners with fear of rolling them over if too much speed was used when negotiating bends. They were quick in a straight line but didn't like stopping, and used more fuel than the Exon Valdez leaked. A quick run transfer to say, London, as was done occasionally, usually meant two stops for fuel on the way down. However, they were exciting to drive and this one was affectionately known as 'The Beast', for obvious reasons.

Our board was now top of the pile meaning we were out next. The phone rang and before I could look up, Jon had covered the quarter mile in the blink of an eye to get to the phone and answer it before it had barely rung. Still seated, I stared at him writing furiously and not saying much, with my thought processes going into overtime. Finally he spoke.

"Ok thanks, that'll be Eagle 4", before replacing the receiver. He briefly looked at me, then grabbing the keys, started walking quickly out of the mess room and down the corridor towards the garage. He started speaking as he left.

"We've got a jumper."

"Fuck", I thought as my heart started to beat out of my chest, and my brain tried to kick into action. One thing experience has taught me, is to never assume and visualise what you are going to. Have a vague trail of thought of what may be going on but don't plan individual actions out because invariably the situation will be different upon arrival, enough to throw and confuse. Even with the experienced guys in the mess room who were unfazed by everything and didn't normally stir from their game of scrabble or cards, would look up at words such as 'jumper' or 'multiple stabbing', and as they did, I caught sight of their gaze, heavily in my direction, as I now quickly walked out of the mess room.

Jon had already decided he was driving and in the seconds it took me to get out into the garage, The Beast was running and revving up, with a cloud of exhaust pluming from the rear. I climbed in and before the door was shut we were off, giving me grief to attempt to put my seat belt on.

The jumper was from a multi-storey car park in the city, only about three miles from station and Jon was in racing driver mode. At the time, I didn't scare easily but his driving was much too fast. With blue lights flashing and sirens wailing, we approached slowing vehicles so quickly that only by luck and not judgement did we not rear end them, and the wrong side of the road saw most of our driving action regardless of whether on-coming vehicles were moving over or not. Then at a small traffic island, he attempted to negotiate it with so much speed, I genuinely thought we were going to roll over, and I'm sure wheels left the ground. Of course, with experience now, it's realised that getting to scene quickly, although important, does not outweigh putting the ambulance crew and the public at risk of injury, and the more adrenaline created in the veins of the crew, the less able they are to do their job when they get there. Only in very rare cases does getting on scene a couple of minutes earlier make a difference to the outcome of the patient.

The glorious sound of that V8 punched through and we neared the scene within minutes, still alive ourselves and still with an unscathed truck. How, I'm still not sure to this day; but we did, and by now I had got so much adrenaline in my system I was shaking. Jon was hyperactive. Turning the final corner, the police, already on scene, had blocked off the road, and seeing The Beast coming at great speed, a young copper quickly moved a traffic cone to one side to allow us through. Before us in the road, alongside the eight story car park was a body of what looked like a male. Alighting The Beast, I cautiously approached it, but Jon beat me, such was his demeanour and excitement. He reminded me of the Duracell Bunny that just keeps going, and never stops. He piped up.

"There's nothing for us to do here. He's dead. "I looked down at the pile of 'mush'. Male clothing adorned legs and arms which lay at grossly deformed angles. Smashed bones stuck out of the skin in a shiny way, glinting with blood, and his torso seemed shorter than it should have been. But it was his head that got to me. It had literally exploded, revealing more bone fragments and brain tissue in a 'squirted' pattern, spraying three feet from the body. It reminded me of fish roe from the chippy; a sort of soft pale pink matter mixed with blood. His face was distorted with one eye being significantly higher than the other and a stare about him that emerged a weird humanoid persona. His jaw was displaced grotesquely to the side with teeth ripped out and any amount more of blood and snot surrounding.

I'd seen the remnants of severe trauma before. One in several bags at the mortuary some months before and the bloke under the train with Chip. As each of these growing cases were dealt with, there was becoming more and more circumstance. Even the poor train guy wasn't out in the open. He'd got a degree of privacy with only part of him poking out into the public area. This jumper was somehow different. He was un camouflaged, in the open, almost vulnerable. Laid out for all to see the grotesque mess of what was left of him. In the other cases it had been a lesson in anatomy. This was here. A real, dead, vile sight of a person, that 20 minutes before had stood somewhere up on the top floor of the car park.

A group of people who'd gathered to gawp at this poor blokes unfortunate ending was being moved on by the police. Jon and I fetched a tarpaulin that ambulances of the time carried so we could cover up the body. But on returning to it, I felt an over whelming nausea flood over me. Not sure whether this was adrenaline, fear or the sight of such trauma at an early stage in my career, but I decided to retire to the relative comfort and privacy of the rear saloon of The Beast. There was nothing we could do here anyway aside of wait until the Police had discharged us from scene. I sat in the back imminently about to vomit, having told Jon where I'd be. I think my facial pallor probably told him I was not at my best. And there I stayed for ten minutes or so until I'd gotten myself together and felt better.

Several days later, the case appeared in the local paper which raised more questions than answers. The deceased male who fell from the top floor of the multi story car park was happily married with children. He had a good job and no medical history including that of mental health. He had been an ordinary man leading an ordinary life and on the day of his death he left for work as normal, kissed the wife and told her he'd see her later. He shouldn't even have been in the location where he died, but some distance away where he worked. There was no evidence on any of the car park floors of a struggle, and being before CCTV, there was no evidence of what had occurred. His car was even still parked where he worked, some 10 miles away, with no one aware that he'd left work, having arrived as he usually did in the morning, with no one noticing he wasn't still there an hour later. A complete mystery. Did he have a secret 'other' life? Was he wrapped up in some money or drug related problem and was executed Mafia style? Certainly many months later the case was not solved.

An eerily similar case occurred a few years later, when I attended a job at the markets in Birmingham. This was a vibrant place between the hours of midnight and 10.00am, and served the traders with fresh veggies, fish, meat and other such goods that were destined to end up in the shops and restaurants later that day. After 10.00am, all washed down, the place became deserted with only the odd car or workman busying themselves. I was by now working on the Paramedic Motorcycle Unit and received a call to attend the markets in the mid afternoon to a report of a collapsed male. Upon arrival the crew had been on scene for a few minutes and were performing CPR on a young guy, I'd guessed was in his late 20's. He was in the middle of a large concreted car park and not near buildings. This place was usually adorned with trucks at night but was now deserted with few if any vehicles near. He was wearing an expensive suit, white shirt and tie and upon my arrival, I didn't see any evidence of trauma, or other clues as to why such a young bloke would be in cardiac arrest at this location. With his upper clothes now removed, CPR continued but we became very aware after about 20 minutes that he was 'ballooning'; severe subcutaneous emphysema is a condition where air enters the subcutaneous tissues around the chest, neck and face, as if someone was pumping air in under pressure, causing the individual to swell, in this case, grotesquely. It was quite obvious that this man had been subject to considerable trauma, and the most likely cause was a vehicle strike, but there were no vehicles around.

Within the next five minutes, the man's face and neck were one big round ball, with his eyes now merely slits and his cheeks blown out, such was the swelling. The result of ventilating him with a bag valve mask. Resuscitation was futile. He was dead. Our attempt ceased, and the police, now on hand, declared this a crime scene. Myself and the crew cleared up our kit, gave our details to the officers and cleared the location.

Several days later, having made a police statement, some very strange details emerged. The deceased's car was found on the top floor of a local multi-story car park, located some two hundred metres from where we had attempted resuscitation upon him. His car was locked with his keys being in his jacket pocket. There was no evidence of which floor he may have jumped from, and none displaying where he may have landed on the floor if indeed he did fall from a height. Forensic testing failed to find evidence of impact with a vehicle, and a post mortem revealed massive chest trauma including a severed aorta, the main blood vessel exiting the heart. This means he would have been unconscious and dead very soon after the trauma, meaning if he had have fallen a height, there was no way he could have walked or crawled to where we found him. There were no witnesses, and a background check on him revealed nothing which might suggest someone deliberately killed him. So, how did he end up where he did, and what was the cause of his trauma? To this day I'm none the wiser.

Most ambos have a particular disliking of a body part; for some its feet, others it might be hands or eyes. For me it's deformed faces in traumatic death. I've seen many, many since then. Such as the poor guy squashed under a ten ton industrial roll of paper, or the teenager hanging out of the speeding car whose head struck a lamp post at speed as the driver lost control. Or the pillion motorcycle rider who was decapitated when they struck barbed wire at speed. These days there is counselling and supportive networks in place to help us all to manage and cope with the after effects of such sights. In the 90's there was none. Piss taking in the mess room with work mates was as near as it got, and must never be under valued. Chatting with others who were there at the time and saw what I saw, with associated 'black' humour, has its place and is documented and written about. This doesn't take away, however, my stress bucket and a wonder if any one of these experiences will invade my nightmares in years to come.

CHAPTER 22. DOORS OF OPPORTUNITY.

West Midlands Ambulance Service led the field in pre hospital innovation. It pioneered the use of paramedic motorcycles to get emergency aid to the patient quicker, and in doing so, was a forerunner for reducing response times; the very core of what all British ambulance services now operate under. From 1989 when the motorcycle project first started, Norton Commanders were used in Coventry and the Black Country. 588cc rotary engined machines, they were quick but suffered some reliability issues of overheating, and were quite dated in design which had the potential for handling problems; something that could not be afforded when riding at speed in the urban setting. The Police had been using them but were phasing them out in favour of the more modern four stroke BMWs. Training for the riders was minimal and the clothing used wasn't the best. The scheme from the start however, had been a success in reducing response times but were an expensive piece of kit per man. And they were grossly under marketed. Then in 1992, tragedy struck when one of the paramedic riders, a brilliant ambassador for the unit, was in collision with a van and was sadly killed on active duty. It was an accident that shouldn't have happened and given the right training I felt could have been avoided. The motorcycle scheme was now seen in a different light; it was dangerous and carried too much risk. It was suspended indefinitely.

I'd been riding bikes since 1985 and had gone on to pass

my advanced motorcycle test with The Institute of Advanced Motorists. From a work perspective I was by 1992 an ambulance technician. I was deeply saddened by the loss of one of our paramedic riders and felt passionate about putting forward some ideas for improvement. So I wrote to the Chief Ambulance Officer Barry Johns, constructively criticising the way the paramedic motorcycle scheme had been run. I'd felt there were many areas for improvement; choice of bike, kit, training, riders, operational jurisdiction and marketing, and the bikes had the potential for advertising and putting the service in a better light. I remember posting the letter and wondering if I'd done more harm than good. I had, after all, constructively, but harshly, criticised the service. This was going to go well.....or I'd have my career cut very short!

About a week later, Barry Johns instructed a senior officer to conduct a review of the paramedic motorcycle scheme. The officer got me in the office and asked me to do all the donkey work of this review, as he knew nothing about bikes. I put forward recommendations following the Police model of clothing, rider selection, choice of bike and training amongst many other ideas. It seemed a simple idea to me to adopt systems that were already in place and proven. I just had to make sure that what may have been utilised would suit the purpose of the paramedic, after all, the role of the police rider was inherently different to that of the medic. We would need to carry much more gear for example, and perhaps wouldn't need to achieve the same speeds. My findings were put into a fancy report by the senior officer, who of course put his name to it and took all the credit. But that was not the issue. What was important to me was that all of my recommendations were adopted and in 1994 the scheme was reintroduced. Late in 1993 I had successfully completed my paramedic course and was invited to apply to become a paramedic biker. My career, and indeed my life, was about to drastically change, as doors would now become open to me that I never dreamed possible.

I completed a police standard motorcycle course in 1994 along with two other successful colleagues and the scheme was relaunched and well marketed now with four riders, using Roy Legge, an existing rider from the scheme's earlier days. Two bikes in the Black Country covering Wolverhampton, Dudley and Walsall, and two of us in Birmingham. The bikes were striped up, visually becoming very high profile and were in the paper and appeared on the television. Myself and Jon 'Wedgey' Wedge covered the whole of the Birmingham area, from the far tip of Four Oaks in Sutton Coldfield in the north, to Longbridge in the south, and everything in between. Response was largely by listening to the radio and self responding to jobs, but as we became better known, crews would ask for the bikes to attend because they could see the advantage of having rapid paramedic support, especially where, at this time, paramedics were still few and far between as most ambulances were manned by technicians. These were similar to paramedics but used a few less drugs and clinical skills.

The rapid response cars were yet to get off the ground. This meant that many of the jobs attended were at the top end of severity and were often life threatening. Stabbings, shootings, road crashes, machinery and factory accidents, building collapses and multiple casualty incidents. We were very proactive and pushed the scheme whenever the opportunity arose, doing school visits and radio interviews. Local businesses got involved and purchased for us Honda's Pan European to add to the fleet. This was, at the time, the latest generation of touring motorcycle that the emergency services were taking up and was to prove very good in our fleet. The project went from strength to strength and although I left it in 1998, my initial input has seen it continue to grow and now even has its own television fly on the wall TV documentary show, 'Emergency Bikers' starring Mark 'Flymo' Hayes, Steve

'Forrest' Harris and Steve 'Harry Potter' Cooper. The bikes, now as then, carry a range of advanced patient equipment, but more importantly, they have the ability to get a paramedic to the scene quickly, often accessing areas that no other vehicle could do, such as shopping centres and canal towpaths.

Scanning and listening in to the ambulance radio became a good way of obtaining work as a bike paramedic; letting the rider decide what jobs might require my assistance, and whether that job was geographically possible to get to. My helmet had radio comms mounted inside, allowing me to sit on the bike parked up somewhere, often centrally in Birmingham, and listen in. The scheme in general though was new and exciting to the public, many thinking we were the police, even though the graphics used on the bikes had been carefully chosen to be different. And when I wasn't sat on the machine, a hand portable radio alerted me to what was going on. The excitement didn't stop with the public. Imagine taking two passions of my life, being a paramedic, and riding motorbikes, then add in a large helping of adrenaline, on-the-edge-of-your-pants action, speed, blood and guts, and you've got a cocktail of what I had for four years. And there wasn't a minute, not one, that I didn't love or would change if I had my time over again. And of course, these four years brought yet more jobs and experiences.

Occasionally this roaming and self responding led to coincidences of attendance, such as the time that, whilst riding along in a southern suburb, I heard a crew being given a cardiac arrest locally to where I happened to be. I hadn't heard the exact address but pulled over to call up and ask, then to write it on the bike's white fuel tank that sat between my knees in chinagraph pencil. Having been given the location, I quickly realised that not only was I already in the road, but I was actually right outside the address. Climbing off the bike and grabbing my bag, I rushed up the garden path and knocked on the door. The lady that opened it still had the phone in her hand, and was still speaking to the ambulance operator. Her jaw dropped at the ferocious speed in which the ambulance service responded to her in her time of need, and was quite speechless for a few seconds with mouth agape. On this occasion, even attending quickly couldn't save the poor man whose heart had stopped. Sometimes, if your time is up, it's up.

Early on, my paramedic motorcycle career found me with my head in the clouds. It was new and exciting, producing more adrenaline than I could shake a stick at, and to think I'd been given a marked up bike, the best gear available, and could basically do what I wanted, when I wanted. I craved for my shifts to start, and dreaded their finish, sometimes taking on extra jobs just to extend the pleasure. I was in heaven, and looking back, very, and I mean, *very* lucky to have been able to experience something which only a handful of people in the world have done. Fewer people have had the pleasure of a job this good.

The icing on the cake on this particular day was the beautiful weather, with light Saturday afternoon traffic reminiscent of 1994. Early afternoon saw me riding in Birmingham city centre. It had been a relatively quiet day, of a 1000hrs until 1900hrs shift, but that didn't matter. It was warm and sunny and the roads were dry. Riding at speed was so much more pleasurable when I knew that tyre grip at speed was better. I'd had a job first thing which saw me ride from Northfield in the south to Chelmsley Wood in the east; a distance of some 10 miles. The call was to a chest pain of cardiac origin, and although the distance was relatively long, the nearest crew at the time of the call had been some miles away and a technician crew of differing clinical ability. So I called it in, and self responded.

The ride was fantastic; bends eaten up with lean until metal contacted tarmac giving the familiar sound of such, facilitating an adjustment of boot position to avoid wearing them away, and the customary smile that only bikers know. Overtakes were executed with hesitation until the opening was clear, at which point the target vehicle was dispensed with. Clear duel carriageways were throttled into, drawing the horizon ever near with a rapidity that made me realise I had the best job in the world. Forward vision and progress was plotted through the traffic, slowing to allow cars to complete their move before taking them on the inside, then overtaking long lines of cars and anticipating drivers plans and movements. Smoothly braking, rapidly accelerating and making that safe progression. And they were paying me for this.

Upon arrival, I was positively buzzing. The bike 'ticked' away as it cooled, the tyres groaned with heat, and the 'chicken strips' on the edge of the tyres were barely visible where I'd had the bike virtually on its side, or so it seemed round the traffic islands and sharper corners. The bike had worked hard and I'd been rewarded with rushes of adrenaline. The crew had been in attendance some few minutes and assessed the patient as not needing my services. A confirmatory check and I said my goodbyes, riding sedately towards the Sutton Coldfield area.

Shifts were worked year round, and although I didn't cover nights, the work rosters were altered to cover the day light hours as the seasons changed. Riding in the heat of a hot summers day did become draining and dehydrating and conversely, the bitter cold of winter brought so many layers of clothing I could hardly move. And the constant threat of ice, the bikers enemy.

Christmas Day 1995 started out much as any other. It was a mild day and I'd left home early leaving the kids who'd already worn out the toys that Santa had brought. A couple of jobs came and went without significance, then while in the city centre, the radio shot forth my Zulu 5 call sign to dispatch me to a stabbing at the railway station. I was local and knew I'd be on scene within minutes so hoped backup wouldn't take too long. British Transport Police are based at the station so I presumed they'd already be on scene, and besides, most stabbings are relatively minor and often turn out to be workmen having cut themselves, or other such occurrences.

I weaved through the light traffic and turned into the car park to head towards the normal emergency vehicle parking bay, and assumed I'd be met by a member of rail staff or police who would take me down to a platform or wherever the patient was.

As I approached the bay, in front of me I saw what looked like a woman lying on her side, motionless and all alone. As I neared she was wearing an Indian sari, and covered in blood. I called 'on scene' and leaving the emergency lights on for some traffic protection, I parked up and jumped off. It was worse than I thought. Even seasoned ambos rarely see massive blood loss. This was one occasion. Not only was she lying in a large pool of blood, but it had run down and across the tarmac in a torrent. There were litres of it.

She was a woman of about 30 I'd guessed, and lay very still with her eyes half open and not breathing. She had multiple stab wounds to her face, arms, throat and torso, and had been attacked in a violent and frenzied way. A quick pulse check revealed nothing, and a connection to my cardiac monitor showed a flat line. I also noticed that the blood around her had congealed enough to make me realise she had been there for long enough to make any attempt at resuscitation futile. Her condition was not compatible with life and she was pronounced dead on scene. What had struck me as strange was that she was all alone; although it had only taken me a few minutes to arrive, there were no police, no public, and nobody at that stage to shed any light on the horrific event. But that soon changed when I called in that I was dealing with a murder. Within minutes, Police were everywhere and the whole place was cordoned off.

As if happening on Christmas Day hadn't been bad enough, when the details emerged, it was worse. The woman's three children had been fatally stabbed some hours before at her home by their father, her husband, who'd proceeded to drive her the 120 miles to Birmingham, where upon he'd chosen the station car park to inflict the same fate, attacking her with ferocity and throwing her out of the car before driving off. The river of blood meant her heart had still been beating as she bled to death, and probably in the early stages was conscious and aware of her injuries. Being Christmas Day, the station was quiet with only a skeleton service operating, so no one witnessed the attack, which had to be recalled on CCTV.

A very tragic end to a whole family. It was believed the motive had been a psychiatric condition on the part of the husband who was shortly tracked down and arrested.

CHAPTER 23. TWO LIVES CUT SHORT.

Donna was the apple of her parent's eye. A lovely 19 year old with looks, motivation and prospects. Achieving four 'A' levels at school, her university phase was mapped out and all seemed good. She'd obtained a job at a local coffee shop where she was popular with both the customers and her colleagues, and such was her demeanour, the owners had wanted her to take over the manager's role which had recently come up, but by this time she had other plans.

Some weeks earlier, a friend had introduced Donna to Darren. She was reluctant to let her parents meet him, and so played down the relationship, even though, as time went on, her mother knew they were getting serious. Donna's parents were well to do; her father was a business man and earned enough to keep them in a large five bedroomed house in a very desirable part of town. Range Rovers and BMWs adorned the gravel driveway, and the family enjoyed two or three foreign holidays a year. He was a Mason, and she was in the Women's Institute, and they were proud of what they'd achieved. Darren on the other hand, represented all that Donna's parents despised; unemployed, no qualifications and no achievements aside of a criminal record for drug and driving offences. He lived with his mother on an undesirable council estate and was the product of the lower social class. Binge drinking, fighting, illegally driving and racing his mates were common pastimes, and his 'working' week consisted of occasional cash in hand labouring jobs on a building site.

Things had started well for Donna in her relationship. She enjoyed the rebellious lifestyle Darren offered her, and after a while decided to introduce him to her mother. Straight away there were problems, and clearly Darren was not liked. Her mother saw him for what he was, but the more she objected, the more Donna rebelled and dug her heels in, even though her relationship with Darren was far from perfect. He'd started threatening her, and his drunken bouts saw her gain the product of his anger. She'd stay away from home long enough for the bruising to subside so there was less explaining to do. And now she found herself pregnant.

With her education waining into the distance, her life revolved around Darren. The two of them had taken on a flat, on the same run down council estate he'd known all his life, and she'd fallen into the lifestyle; the dog on the balcony, the latest television, wearing stolen top brand clothing, and not two pennies to rub together aside of what little Darren gave her for food, and what he spent down at the pub from his cash in hand jobs and deals on the side. She still saw her mother from time to time, who reeled in anguish at what had become of her promising girl. And of course the impending baby added to the difficulties. But as the pregnancy progressed Donna found her relationship with her mother improving and her mother responded with mellowing towards the situation, even inviting Darren over for tea, in a bid to win her back.

The weeks went by and the birthdate neared with no sign of a labour starting. Donna attended the antenatal clinic on the expected date with the result that the baby was stubbornly staying put. On this Saturday, Darren was in the pub, so Donna had been to see the midwife with her friend and had persuaded Darren to pick her up after the appointment which he had reluctantly agreed to do. Saturday afternoons were for drinking with mates and watching the football on the big screen in the bar, not for picking up the girlfriend who was heavily pregnant and now carrying bags of shopping. She got into the car and unable to wear her seatbelt due to her condition, they headed off.

What happened next is unclear and was never able to be proven, but eye witnesses reported seeing the car weaving at speed from one side of the road to the other in a well to do suburban road. The car lost control, and collided hard with the corner of a garden wall, striking the front of the car on the passenger side. A fire started, and within seconds was spreading. Motorists stopped to render assistance and someone ran into the hotel for help. Staff appeared soon after with fire extinguishers spraying them at the fire. Householders came out of the houses to greet commotion and excitement. Many stood helpless as the two occupants of the crushed, mangled wreck screamed for help. One lady scooped water from a front garden pond to throw it on the growing inferno. The crying, shouting and piercing screams from the car became more panicky, but the fire was beating the helpers back, the pitiful shouts and cries from the passenger side quickly became less, then stopped. Darren, trapped and still screaming, managed to get his top half out of the drivers window and created a gap between him and the flames. His shouts cut the air even over the top of the rest of the commotion, as on lookers, neighbours, and hotel staff buzzed around, still fighting the fire, which by now they were getting the better of.

Within seconds of the impact, a 999 call had been made asking for ambulance, police and fire services. As the call was given out over the police airwaves, two motorcycle police officers were, by coincidence passing the far end of the road, picked up on the job and got to the scene within 60 seconds as the fire was beginning to become under control. They used their bike fire extinguishers to finally douse the flames. What they saw through the smoke, shocked them to the core. The call to me came through at a similar time to the bike cops, although I was slightly further away but already heading in the direction. My helmet spoke up.

"Metro Zulu 5, Zulu 5, you receiving over?" The adrenaline started seeping into my veins, quickening my pulse and breathing as it always did when I knew a job was on the cards. I pressed the button on the handle bar.

"Zulu 5 go ahead over".

"Zulu 5 can we get you running please to an RTA persons trapped?" Replied Metro. Now the adrenaline went ballistic and I could feel my heart beating as I got myself prepared to set off. Control gave me the location and I switched on the blue emergency lights before a quick mirror and shoulder check then off I headed. Within minutes I turned into the road where I was met by a police car with flashing blue roof lights blocking the road. Negotiating around it, I continued on.

The incident lay in front of me to the left of the road and over the pavement. I pulled up short, flicked out the side stand, and leaning the bike onto it, killed the engine. I knew this road to be busy, and loud with buses, lorries, cars, cyclists and chattering children. Tree lined, there was always a chorus of birdsong. But now there was nothing, and aside of the screams there was the same silence I'd heard before. The silence which implied death of the mutilation and horrible variety. What had been a sports type car had collided with a wall at what looked like some considerable speed. An ambulance crew had pulled up to the scene a few minutes before me and were holding and supporting a male whose upper body was hanging out of the drivers window.

I lifted my gear off the bike and stood momentarily at the passenger front door of the car to survey what was going on, and more importantly what my plans were going to be as the only paramedic on scene. The car initially struck me as odd. It was shorter than it should have been, the wheels having been pushed significantly back by the force of the impact. The front of the car was completely burnt out as far back as, and including the front passenger seat, and all that remained of the bonnet was a mass of smouldering, crumpled and paintless metal. The rear of the car was untouched, and the paint gleamed in contrast with the front. This fire had been explosive and intoxicating, and had clearly taken hold very quickly. The front passenger seat was covered in a tarpaulin sheet with the shape of a person underneath. It was motionless and a quick lift of it revealed a body, distinguishable as one but burnt beyond recognition. No hair, no skin, no pink colouring; just blackened and charred flesh and so obviously deceased as to require no further confirmation but this initial visual check. I replaced the sheet and turned my attention to the driver, who after a check in the back of the car, appeared to be the only other occupant. His naked torso was out of the car and I could see some obvious and severe burns down his left side. Abuse was being hurtled at the guys who were supporting him, with a real tone of panic.

"Come on, hurry up. Get me out of this fuckin' car.......agggghhhhhhhhhh don't touch me there you fuckin' wanker. Gi' me somethin' for the fuckin' pain man....." He was a young guy, I'd guessed about early twenties, with loads of unmatching tattoos and a shaven head. My immediate impression of him was that if I'd walked past him in the street, I wouldn't look him in the eye for fear of getting the 'who the fuck you lookin' at?' treatment, dare I stereo type, but I'm sure you get the idea. But now this didn't matter. I'm a Health Care Professional and he was about to become my patient regardless.

The air was heavy with the pungent smell of acrid smoke and burning rubber, which etched into my nostrils as I made my way towards the noise. I knew that creating a rapport with this patient was going to be difficult, and after some calming reassurance I got a first name of Darren. Patients who experience pain will often present as rude and demanding, and this guy was no exception, giving me a fair bit of expletive before revealing his name, but his need for pain relief was obvious. I'd estimated he had 1st, 2nd and 3rd degree burns to a large part of the left side side of his torso, left arm, left shoulder, and left side of his face, and following assessment, an oxygen mask was placed over his face and a cannula was inserted into his arm for some intravenous fluids to be given. At the time, Entonox, or 'gas and air' was my only form of pain relief, and had been given early by the ambulance crew but wasn't effective with Darren and had been stopped, so I was fairly relieved when the roving medic arrived to give something which would be more effective. These were doctors who worked with the ambulance service to provide a greater depth of clinical care than I could give to cases such as these.

As Dr Jon took over the lead clinical care, I found myself standing on the bonnet, acting as a drip stand holding the bag of intravenous fluid that was now attached to the patient's arm. It was a rare commodity to have the luxury and opportunity of being able to view the scene with a fair degree of detail, as on most occasions, as the lead clinician, I would have been far too busy sorting the casualty out. I looked at things with my detective cap on and tried to piece together in my head the sequence of events. Striated tyre marks on the road going back some distance implied the car had slid sideways with speed and a loss of control, slewing the car left and right before the collision with the corner of the brick wall, predominantly on the passenger side. The wall held back a lawn on a sloping driveway of a plush detached house, and as such did not give upon impact proving to be a solid, strong structure.

The engine has been pushed backwards towards the occupants, causing the front seat passenger to take most of the impact. The bonnet was crumbled, and even with thick soled bike boots on, was warm under foot as I stood on it, shuffling around trying to balance on the bent edges. It brought home the realisation of just how hot and ferocious this fire had been. Wispy smoke still rose and after some time nausea set in, as I continued to survey with my birds eye view. The steering wheel, half of which was just a burnt steel ring, had deformed in and upwards, and the windscreen had either popped out or been removed. Plastic dash lay grossly distorted and smashed, and the gear lever was nearly in the back seat, which was strewn with empty drinks cans and rubbish. From where I was standing Darren's legs were not visible, but the lack of leg room made me suspect that he probably had lower limb fractures to complicate his burns.

The patients shouting and foul language subsided as intravenous pain relief from the doctor started to settle him as the Fire Service worked tirelessly using hydraulic cutting gear and skill, and within half an hour, the roof and side of the car had been removed and Darren was released. His burns already dressed, he was placed into spinal immobilisation and onto the waiting stretcher by the other ambulance guys, and with a police motorcycle escort, the ambulance raced off with lights and two tone horns towards the hospital with the doctor in the back, and as the familiar ambulance sound faded into the distance, I cleared up my gear and returned the pannier to the bike. By now the whole area had been cordoned off and the police investigative teams started to examine the scene properly, in order to determine just what had happened.

The area had initially been screened off to prevent onlookers from visualising the horror. Now, there was an eery silence. It's somewhat indescribable and very strange where the silence is almost deafening. So prominent as to be out of place. And so representative of hideous death.

All of the rushed, acute care had gone. No more ambulance or doctor. Just people with measuring tapes, instruments and forensic cameras. The Fire service were clearing up and generally helping, and once the public had been moved on, removed the tarpaulin off the body. Only now was the full horror of the accident revealed. The body was charred black beyond most recognition of identity, and initially I couldn't even work out if I was looking at a man or a woman. Then the large protruding abdomen confirmed to me this was a heavily pregnant female. Her lips were four times the size and her tongue also, protruding out beyond her mouth. Her eyes were shut and all trace of hair had gone. She'd died in the position she was last in; leaned forward left hand wrapped around the A pillar, right hand flat against the dashboard. She knew what was coming and had braced herself. But bracing alone wouldn't save her or her unborn child. Looking down, her legs had received the same fate. Cloth had been incinerated away, revealing bare legs, charred, blackened and burnt, and fixed in the brace position. I looked at her and imagined what had been going through her mind seconds before the impact. Try as I did not to, my human instinct made me consider the emotive. 30 years on, thoughts of this image still flicker across my mind. Dulled down somewhat, but still there. Another few drops of water into the bucket.

The inquest was held several months later. Commendation was given by the Coroner to the two motorcycle police officers who undoubtedly saved the life of the driver by putting out the remainder of the fire, as well as to the hotel staff and the members of the public who did their bit. The police were sure there was a case of dangerous or reckless driving on the part of the driver, based upon eye witness reports, but there was insufficient evidence to prove it. In disgust by the attendees to the inquest, Darren turned up with his new girlfriend, now heavily pregnant. As if that doesn't stereo type the sort of person he was. Donna's mother was later unsuccessful in filing a private prosecution against Darren, and now has to live with the loss of her daughter and unborn grandchild in such tragic circumstances.

CHAPTER 24. SOMETIMES, YOUR TIME IS UP......AND SOMETIMES IT'S NOT.

None of us can accurately predict what will happen during our days as we go about our business. Of course, we can have a say in some elements, but there are just too many variables to know if we are going to collide with a truck, or get stabbed standing in the queue at the supermarket. Fortunately for most of us the latter two rarely, if ever, happen. Which means of course, that 99.99% of the thousands of patients I've attended over the years, woke up on any particular morning without knowing that at some point during the day my path would cross with theirs. Aside perhaps of the chronically ill individual, or the failed suicide that would both know some time before that they would likely end up at my door. And as if circumstance hadn't dealt them enough of a blow, fate would also have a say as to the severity of illness or injury that would befall them. It therefore never fails to amaze me the level of trauma that the human body can be subjected to, for the individual to simply stand, brush themselves down, and walk away. Conversely it is the opposite; such as the poor middle aged lady who tripped up a raised paving slab in a busy street in Birmingham, to land on both knees heavily, receiving compound fracture to both femurs and bleeding to death before help could arrive.

Ernest Bryant, 80, and his 76 year old wife, Phyllis, had been planning a trip to her sister's for some months. It was a fair distance from their home in Coventry, to Maud and Harry's place in The Lake District, and had needed a fair bit of thought on Ernie's part. He was a tall, dapper man of some six feet in height, with dark combed Brylcreamed hair and a wispy trimmed moustache. Always smartly dressed, he kept good health by walking several miles a week, and had never smoked, and only drinking alcohol occasionally on high days and holidays. His relationship with his wife was very one sided; he was obsessively dominant, she reluctantly submissive, and that's the way it had always been. He had the first and final word, and her ideas were little more than just that, which invariably fell on deaf ears. Phyllis also fitted the description of smart, wearing her pinny around the house to keep her dress clean whilst going about her wifely duties. Her health had been in decline for some years, with arthritis, and now more recently developing a heart complaint, both of which saw her heavily medicated. She did however love her husband with devotion and passion, and in return, Ernie too, loved her, and cared for her.

Their forthcoming few days away, were to be the longest they'd driven for some time, and Ernie made sure that everything was checked to reduce the risk of incident. His years spent as a cabinet maker, made him fastidious and meticulous for detail. He confirmed the route, the exact distance, how much fuel they would likely use, and what the cost would be. His Peugeot was 10 years old, but he'd bought it new and looked after it, washing it regularly on Sunday mornings between 8 and 9am, and having it serviced on the dot, every six months, even though nowadays, they did very little relative mileage. In his former years, Ernie had done his own vehicle maintenance, but as he'd become older, although still fit and active, he'd decided to let the younger blokes do his oil changes and servicing. So for the journey ahead, he had the car checked over by the garage and was happy that all things seemed right. He packed the car the day before and early on the Saturday morning, they set off.

It had been decided at the last minute, that they would take Minnie with them. Born Rose Minerva Hobson in December 1928, as Phylis's youngest cousin, she was nick named Minnie, after Minnie Mouse, created a month earlier by Walt Disney. And so the name stuck. She'd never married, and had worked all her life for the same insurance company in the offices until the firm folded a few years earlier and she took retirement. She'd never driven, and had always been fiercely independent. But since her leaving work she had taken to become confused and increasingly forgetful and withdrawn and her GP had diagnosed Alzheimers Disease. She was still able to live largely alone though, aside of a home help who came in five days a week.

The late change of plans had annoyed Ernie. It had upset his schedule but Phyllis had suggested the idea they take her, and despite his reservations he knew how much it meant to her, so he agreed. Minnie had stayed the night with them on the Friday, and with some cajoling on the Saturday morning to get ready, finally they set off, Minnie in the back of the car and Phyllis sitting in the front passenger seat.

Phyllis was a nervous passenger, and feared the motorway with its levels of traffic and congestion. She'd seen a decline in Ernie's eyesight and reaction time with his driving over the last few years, and this had been one reason why their journeys now only really consisted of weekly trips to the shops and bingo on a Thursday. She'd suggested taking the train, but Ernie had rejected the idea as stupid, as they would need transport in the wilds of Cumbria. Phyllis suspected that his decision was part of the bravado to prove to himself he still had what it took to drive that far. And being the ever obedient wife, she bowed down and accepted his word. None the less, they were both looking forward to a few days away in The Lakes to spend some time with Maud and Harry, whom they'd not seen for several years, as Harry was now blind and Maud didn't drive.

7am saw them negotiate the short drive to the M6, and on northwards they went. Traffic was light which pleased Phyllis, and the sun was shining. Idle talk wasn't something Ernie practised, despite his wife loving to chat, so they sat in relative silence, with just the occasional comment from her as to the pleasant surroundings, or how happy she felt. Minnie would occasionally say something which was totally unconnected with the journey and Phyllis would humour her with an answer. Ernie gave little in the way of conversation but instead passed his own infrequent comment of how fast other drivers were, or why trucks needed to occupy a certain lane for so long. He wasn't after reply; only to make rhetorical conversation. Phyllis, after all, wasn't capable of vehicular discussion. In Ernie's eyes her topics of chat would be confined to 'female' pastimes, such as cooking, sewing, or by the goodness of his generosity, her bingo trips.

So all was well. The sun was radiant, everything had been checked, and rechecked. They'd set off on time, and were destined northbound to arrive in some three hours time. But fate had decided on this day, to intervene. The Lakes, and a trip up north was not now on the cards, and Maud and Harry were going to be disappointed. A short distance after entering the motorway, the car started misfiring and running a little rough. Ernie ignored it to start with, after all, it had been checked and couldn't possibly go wrong. But it worsened. And now, vibration and shuddering in the car alerted Phyllis, who looked over at her husband with an anxious look. He remained looking forward, even though he was now aware of his wife's fear. Having recently overtaken a slower truck, the Peugeot was now in lane two travelling at about 70mph, but as the shuddering worsened so the car slowed, and Ernie's concentration was now in his own world rather than that around him. He vocalised his thoughts.

"What in the blazes.....," and "I don't believe this. Stan was adamant the car would get us to your sister's". But his own little world did not include vehicles approaching them from behind. It also didn't include trying to get them into lane one, and then onto the relative safety of the hard shoulder. And as a basic safety element, it also didn't include putting on the hazard warning lights. Despite the traffic being very light, as they slowed, cars passed them at a faster and faster rate of speed, and by now Phyllis started voicing her concern.

"What's happening Ernest? Is everything alright?" The fear in her voice was obvious, but rather than words of reassurance, she was greeted with a condescending tone.

"Shut up woman, can't you see I'm trying to sort this?", he shouted, which only served to heighten his wife's terror that she was by now clearly displaying.

Then the shuddering stopped, the ignition lights all came on, and now the car slowed dramatically until it came to a complete stand still. In lane two. Phyllis panicked and started screaming. Her every fear of the motorway was now realised. Stationary in the middle of it with cars passing on either side, some blaring their horns as if the unfortunate couple had elected to stop to admire the scenery. Ernie wasn't panicking. He was annoyed, and started muttering to himself, still completely oblivious to both his surroundings, and the danger they were clearly in. He went for the key, turning it with some force. The engine turned over and over, but not an ounce of life came forth. It didn't fire, and it didn't start. As if fate's loading wasn't enough, the following events were beyond belief; beyond normal comprehension. Ernie pulled the bonnet lever, took off his belt, and opened the door. He walked around the front of the car to the sound of his wife's agonising shouts.

"NO ERNEST, NO. PLEASE GET BACK IN THE CAR.......ERNEST! ERNEST!" Lifting the bonnet, he remained oblivious to her pleading, and her cries. And to the approaching cars. Having some mechanical knowledge, he thought he'd go for the points, and proceeded to remove the distributor cap, with a sort of calmness that one sees when having a lazy Sunday afternoon doing a little tinkering with the engine. All that was missing was a lit pipe, and a mug of steaming tea to complete the picture. But the reality was so very far from this mental image. Despite the traffic still being relatively light, the inevitable was drawing closer. Fate's hand was about to play its ace, and in the blink of an eye, the sound of a rapidly approaching skid quietened Phyllis. For that split second, she silenced. And that silence hit Ernie, pulling him with lightening speed into reality. He rapidly pondered how stupid he'd been, and in retrospect, asked himself the question of why he hadn't tried to get to the hard shoulder. The consequences of his actions were about to become all too clear. The momentary screeching noise of the skid from behind stopped and Ernest braced himself for an impact that he knew would kill him. And with the raised bonnet obstructing his view of what was impending there was nothing he could now do. There was nowhere to go. Then the sound of a car swerving around the rear, made him breathe a sigh of relief as a car passed them on the inside, travelling fairly slowly, clearly having been able to avoid the collision.

Heading northbound on the same sunny morning was Shaun Flynn. Shaun was a traveller who owned and ran a successful roads maintenance business. He drove a transit pickup, and on this morning, was driving just a couple of junctions en route to a job. He'd been pleased that traffic had been light and was planning his job tasks for that day, when he was suddenly, and without warning presented with the car in front braking so hard, he'd locked all four wheels at speed before the brake lights went out, and the car violently swerved to the left. Shaun had been travelling at about 70mph in lane two and never even had reaction time to apply the brakes before he was aware of what was happening. The swerving car, now out of the way, revealed a stationary blue saloon car with the bonnet up, right in his path. He hit it before he could even take his foot off the accelerator, and rammed the Peugeot with massive force, sending it forwards with such ferocity, that by the time the transit had come to a halt, Ernie's car was some 50 metres ahead, and had now veered across to lane three and had collided with the central reservation and was now facing 180 degrees to its original direction and pointing back towards the way it had come.

Shocked and stunned at what had befallen him, Shaun remained motionless for several seconds, trying to take in what had just happened. He shook himself into reality and quickly became aware, that he too, was now stationary in lane two, and a sitting duck. He glanced in his mirror and noticed the traffic behind was slowing to a stop. Severe pain in his neck prevented him from turning his head as he stepped from the van and surveyed the scene. His bonnet was crumpled and folded up towards the smashed windscreen. Exploded headlights and what was left of the front bumper lay on the carriageway. Steam erupted from the front and water poured all over the road. He rotated his body towards the Peugeot and walked towards it, fearful of what he would see. He'd expected, and hoped, that someone would step from it, get out and brush themselves off and it would all be ok. No one would be injured and he could relax. But somehow he knew that wasn't going to be the case. As he approached, the damage was extensive. The back of the car was caved in as far as the back of the front seats. He could see someone in the passenger seat, that the hair said was a female, but she wasn't moving. As he rounded the front, he got a better look at her. There wasn't any visible blood but her head had fallen forward and she remained motionless, with the seat belt still in situ.

Other occupants from the now stationary following cars had walked forwards to the scene, and questions were asked of the driver's whereabouts. Someone suggested he'd walked along the hard shoulder to use the emergency telephone which explained his absence. But a commotion someway behind Shaun's van held the truth. Some distance back along the carriageway, lay a tall elderly male. The impact caused the front of his car to make contact with him, sending him forwards with incredible force and causing him to land supine on the road, to then have his own car go over the top of him traversing down its centre, followed by the Transit van, whose wheels also went either side of him, leaving him pretty much in the centre of the carriageway, and narrowly avoided by the braking vehicles following.

It was unusual for me as a paramedic motorcyclist to be sent to cases on the motorway network as it had been deemed as being too risky, what with the speed and volume of the traffic. However, in the absence of any other available vehicles, I was all they had, and as a case of the lesser of two evils, I was responded.

Sat on the side of the road in a northern suburb, my radio alerted my senses.

"Zulu 5, can you respond please, RTA junction five to six northbound, car verses pedestrian. No ambulance available at this stage, but Medic 11 responding from Solihull over." I acknowledged receipt and thought of my route for a second. As the crow flies, I could virtually see the accident scene, but I needed to access the motorway from an emergency services access point just south of junction five to save having to go all the way to junction four as there was no northbound access at junction five, only an exit. This would take a while but I decided on my route and set off. As a driver of an emergency vehicle responding under blue lights, I concentrated on my riding rather than what I perceived I'd be faced with. There is a need to concentrate on the task at hand of getting there safely, and this is particularly important riding a high powered motorcycle, where the speeds and stakes are higher, especially as it always seemed that everyone was out to get me.

With the sirens screaming, traffic was safely dispensed with time after time as the dynamic process of riding at speed got underway. Forward vision, early riding plans, good use of hesitation, and discretion being the better part valour, saw me enter the motorway, some three miles south of the incident. Motorways can be one of the safest places to ride provided the traffic is flowing, and in the same general direction. So this initially afforded me the opportunity to gain some ground quickly. Within a short space of time, the slowing and queuing traffic signalled I wasn't too far from my patient, and negotiating around the stationary lines of traffic, I came to the front of the line, to be met by a group of people standing around something in the road resembling a body, and some badly damaged vehicles about 50 or 60 metres further ahead.

Before I could alight my bike, a middle aged, frumpy woman with short hair approached me, and with a confident, almost arrogant tone, started to tell me what had happened. With a helmet on and traffic noise from the southbound carriageway, I couldn't hear a word, but her outstretched arms, pointing finger and moving lips told me she had a story to tell of the events. I removed my lid after climbing off the bike and started to get a feel for the scene. Now one thing I'm particularly inept at, is multi tasking on a general scale. You know the sort of thing; making the kids tea, while opening the mail from the morning post, and planning a dinner party for the weekend.

Not a hope. At work, however it's different. In this arena, I have to survey, process information, communicate, triage, treat, direct, consider and command. And boy can that be challenging when you're all alone!

I apologised and asked the woman to repeat herself. So following the cursory frown, sigh, hesitation, upward eye roll and tut, she started again. What we as paramedics at these types of incidents require, is a succinct over view. As valuable as the history of the event is, time spent listening only, could be an airway that's occluding, or a wound that's hosing out. I needed to get into the thick of the scene fast to give the Comms centre a situation report (known as as 'sitrep') of exactly where we were, what type of incident I was dealing with, what dangers were present, and where subsequent resources needed to access, a head count of all casualties, and finally what other services were needed. The woman appeared condescending, like I was a miss-behaving school child, but continued with her account. I, on the other hand, had made up my mind to ignore her around about the second sentence.

".......So I'd said to Malcolm, my husband, not to pack the boot so full as I couldn't get the lid down, and......." At this point she clearly wasn't useful to me and I started to ignore her as other visual information and conclusions were coming in. I knew things were going to be awkward with her when I became aware of a stop mid sentence, a pause, then as I was hurrying away, a question in a raised voice.

"Are you listening to me young man? I used to be a school nurse you know. So I know what I'm talking about.......". She slipped from my attention. I had too much on my plate.

I hurried towards the body in the road where I saw a tall slim elderly man with a face full of abrasions, wearing dirty, abraded trousers revealing bloody skin and raw flesh. His once immaculate shirt, struggled to cover his upper body and the remnants of a brown cloth tie hung loose and precariously at his throat. His degree of consciousness revealed agitation and a sort of 'spaced out' appearance, as he tried to get up off the tarmac but was held down and reassured by the people around him who'd gotten out of their cars to help. I momentarily stooped down to examine him, looking into his eyes. His vacant stare meant he was somewhere else, muttering without making much sense, aside of catching the occasional word.

"Phyllis......Phy....". The words petering out as he drifted. His left arm was partly   de-gloved; the flesh traumatically stripped off revealing the silvery, bloody bone underneath, smashed and at an irregular angle, with blood surrounding it on the bitumen.

Blood on a solid, non absorbent surface such as tarmac can appear to be a huge amount, but often isn't if you can discount it having soaked into clothing. The man's blood loss didn't appear catastrophic but it's never a very good sign if an injury this severe doesn't make an obvious impact on a patient, and often signifies head or spinal injuries, particularly in the presence of agitation such as this man displayed.

One weakness that pre hospital inexperience breeds, is looking at a horrendous injury, or some poor smashed up individual at the scene of a multi casualty incident and stopping to treat when you're first on scene. It's happened to all of us at some stage, and don't let anyone who's worked in this sort of environment say they haven't. They're lying. It's the most difficult thing in the world, as a provider of paramedicine, compassion, love, care and understanding, to stoop at the head of someone's loved one, then get up and leave with only having dished a few words to the bystanders, and maybe a reassuring sentence to the patient. Aside of haemorrhaging severely or an occluded airway that can be rectified simply, a sitrep to Comms at the earliest possible time will save more lives than me spending my time at that point with this one man. And that sitrep can only be done with the information already described.

"Oh thank God you're here", said a guy kneeling alongside the patient, holding his uninjured arm. "This bloke's been run over by that van there", pointing with a directional nod to a vehicle further up the carriageway from us. "It went clean over him, an' spat him out the back". He wasn't bleeding badly and I was happy to leave him in the care of those around him. I looked the patient in the eye again, and with a gentle tone tried to reassure him.

"Don't worry, we'll soon have you sorted. These good people will take care of you for a while." He didn't move his open eyes to meet mine, and I doubted he'd heard or understood me, but one thing I learned a long time ago, is always speak to people, no matter if they can or cannot hear what I'm saying. They just might. I looked up at those nearest to him, and continued, as I rose to my feet, "Guys, you're doing a fantastic job. Keep it going for a bit and I'll be back". They protested as I furthered from them, and I caught the tail end.

"Where ya goin……?" I briefly pondered their frustration at the presentation to a paramedic of an old man completely run over on a motorway with the potential of horrendous injury, only for the medic to compliment them on their actions and then walk away. But it was how we do things. Maybe there were more casualties, and I needed to find them. One down, and counting.

The scene was beginning to tell a story. What I wasn't sure of, was how come a pedestrian was in the carriageway to get run over in the first place, but I reckoned the answer lay in the vehicles up ahead. I hurried on without running and upon arrival at a white transit pickup, looked inside the crumpled cab to see a dusty, untidy interior with a generous littering of empty drink cans and cigarette packets. But no people. A short distance from it was a man standing in lane 3 with his back to me and holding his neck with one hand, and a roll up in the other. As I neared he became aware of someone approaching and turned round. He was a bloke of about 40 I reckoned, rough shaven and looked like he was no stranger to hard labour. I struck first as I approached.

"Hello mate, were you the driver of the Transit?".

"Yes mate," he replied in a gruff Irish tone. "Me feckin' necks killing me". He'd a soft, slightly Southern Irish accent, reminiscent of the travelling community, and he became my second casualty, another that I also wasn't going to stay with at that time.

"Ok, I need you to lie down on the floor to rest your neck and keep it nice and still for me and I'll be back in a minute". He looked taken aback.

"Jasus, I'll not be loyin' on no tarmac. This coat cost me a feckin' fortune". The irony of a man who prioritised on his suede jacket over a potential broken neck. Especially when clearly, the jacket looked like it had been used for laying tarmac, roofing and digging the garden.

"Well just try to keep still then will you? And for Christ's sake don't light that cigarette, or we'll all go up." He looked at me with his head slightly cocked.

"Huh? Oh the ciggy? Yeah no problem. Oil have it later," before popping the grubby roll up behind his ear. Joe public often light up or try to light up a smoke after having had an accident without realising the potential. It's always been automatic with me to instil a 'no light up' or 'put it out' regime at car accidents and although I knew the request to keep still would fall on deaf ears, I hoped he'd listen about not lighting up. My reconnaissance wasn't finished, and I continued on.

Some way in front of the white van, a blue car sat facing me. It resembled one which had picked a fight with a train at a level crossing. The bonnet and general front end was moderately damaged, but I measured damage severity levels in whether I could still tell the make and model. And this was a Peugeot. A good start. And there it ended. For there was no rear end to this car. The remains of the rear number plate sat where the back of the front seats should have been, forced in and crushed by some incredible kinematic forces. The rear wheels had been pushed under the car, and the whole floor pan resembled the shape of a banana, bowed like some speedway 'funny' car of the 1970's. The air was heavy with the smell of petrol, and I suddenly realised I'd been walking across a huge spill. It's often after these sort of jobs that hindsight becomes a wonderful thing. The text books tell us not to enter any scene until safe to do so, which is of course correct. Nobody needs a dead paramedic. But dynamic risk assessment is easier done in hindsight than reality, and I was bloody glad I'd asked the Irish guy not to light up. The windscreen was badly smashed and I couldn't see through it from the front to see if the car was empty or had someone in it from this angle. I walked around and peered in through the driver's window. In the passenger seat was an elderly woman crushed between a sandwich of crumpled metal behind the back of her seat, and the dashboard. Her face was beetroot purple and covered in a fine layer of powdered glass where the windscreen had exploded. Her tongue had been forced out of her mouth and nearly bitten off by the sheer force that snapped her jaw shut, and her head lay at a grossly strange angle that only a broken and probably severed cervical spine would allow. Her partly open eyes stared downwards. All I could think of was how quick this poor lady's death would have been.

I'd been on scene approximately 3 minutes, and gathered all the information I needed for my sitrep. I had a 2 car RTC M6 northbound at junction six, with two serious casualties, and 1 fatality. Access was at the emergency entrance Collector

Road Castle Bromwich onto the northbound carriageway, ambulances to make two, and Police and Fire Service to attend as well as Medic 11 to continue from Solihull. If the air ambulance was available it too should be mobilised. My adrenaline was making me buzz, and now in possession of the facts, I could go and treat.

It's at times like these that making the best use of available resources is paramount. I may not have carried much on the motorcycle then, but a quick shouted request to all the gawping motorists standing with their arms folded watching the show brought forward a plethora of kit. First aid supplies, blankets, fire extinguishers, and tools. If the Fire boys weren't going to be with us for several more minutes, I wanted to make damn sure we'd got at least some means of protection if it went tits up. The Police arrived and between us we managed to utilise a road sign as a make shift spinal board to get my van driver off his feet and away from fire risk, and Ernie was kept warm and cushioned with blanket rolls and jackets. Sadly of course, none of the resources were needed on his poor wife except for a canvas sheet that a truck driver had donated.

Within minutes, the Fire Service and Medic 11 arrived, followed by my ambulances and the two patients were assessed, packaged and transported. The helicopter's ETA was too long and it was decided that the doctor would travel with Ernie and the other paramedic crew would take Mr Flynn. The deceased female becomes the domain of the Coroners Office, and the Police, and as such, due to the scene being one of a crime issue until otherwise proven, the ambulance service has nothing more to do with the body. Nowadays Paramedics can legally pronounce and confirm death has occurred, but at this time of the early 90's, only a doctor could do so, and indeed had done so with a fleeting look. Her injuries were clearly incompatible with life and death was declared.

Before resuming the helmet and riding off, as the motorway

remained shut I went for a proper look at the wreckage and the blue Peugeot shrouded in canvas sheeting from the Fire Service. Why do we do this? Well there are several reasons; we need to get a feel for the kinematics of trauma; that is, the forces inflicted upon the occupants of a vehicle following collision. This is particularly important where there are survivors to add another piece of the jigsaw of potential injuries. Where there is time, and it's appropriate, we do it for the interest of seeing just what damage has been inflicted upon the deceased, and lastly, as a final check to make sure we haven't missed anything......or any one. As I looked behind the front seats, into the crushed mass of unrecognisable steel and plastic, I saw it. The clue which told me there was more than one body in the car. The edge of a hand, quite low down and not very visible. Clearly, very deceased, given the amount of room her body occupied. She had submarined partly under the front seat of her cousin, only to have the floor come up and crush her, as well as the rear of the car violently moving forward. She did not stand a chance.

I left the scene, and the Police and Fire Service had the grisly task of retrieving the bodies from the wreckage and to confirm there were no more in there. The full details of this tragic incident came out some time later at the Coroners inquest. Ernest Bryant survived the accident, and for more than the minimum time required for his subsequent death to not be classified as being as a result of this accident. He sustained brain damage, a fractured pelvis, leg fractures and some internal bleeding. His arm was electively amputated, and he stayed in hospital until he transferred some months later to a nursing home, where he passed away peacefully 12 months later. I don't like to think of the potential torture he may have endured during his final time on this earth of the circumstances of his wife and her cousin's deaths, and hope he survived cocooned in his own little world, oblivious to his actions on that fated day. Shaun Flynn suffered a stable C5,C6 and C7 spinal fracture and made a full recovery.

In conclusion, I never fail to be amazed at what the human body is capable of withstanding. The forces subjected to Phyllis and Minnie were always going to be unsurvivable, and the circumstances of Ernie's injuries should have dictated certain death for him. To be struck by the front of his car whilst standing right up against it, jettisoned forward with immense force, then run over by not one, but two vehicles and spat out of the back, should have caused fatal injuries, and normal mortals would not have survived that degree of trauma. But somehow he did. God clearly wasn't ready for him just yet.

These memories and others feed my bucket. You know, the bucket we all carry around with us, placing into it all the worries, emotions, sights, smells, memories, thoughts and feelings that we pick up on our journey through life. Into my bucket, I placed the trauma of the two ladies, the sight of their squashed bodies, the face of Phyllis, Minnie's crushed fingers barely making an appearance, Ernie's de-gloved arm, and how I could also have become a statistic if my carpet of petrol had ignited. In they went along with many more years worth of 'Ernies'. My bucket is pretty full, and one of these days it will overflow. Sometimes I feel it already has, then I realise, that if I give the bucket a shake, it'll make room for some more. But, having reached middle age, and starting the journey towards retirement, I've discovered ways to take some of the contents out of the bucket; gardening, restoring old cars, shooting, walking, and my dog. Ah, my faithful friend Bessie. Obedient, faithful, comforting, and always by my side. She's probably taken more out of the bucket than anything else (ironically, Bess, alive at the time of writing in 2014, was run over and killed a few years later). It worries me, and the thousands of us all who live stressful lives, that the bigger the bucket, and the more there is in it, the bigger the bang when it goes off. Is it that our foci elsewhere reduces the level in the bucket, or just gives us the ability to squash more in?

"You must see some sights in your job. What's the worst thing you've ever seen?" The question that every paramedic has been asked on many occasions. If I had a dollar for every time someone had asked me that one, I'd be a wealthy man. I always answered it in a modest tone.

"Oh I don't know. I'm sure factory workers and secretaries have elements in their job that are distasteful" I'd say. But they weren't referring to something they thought was distasteful in my world. What they really wanted was a full description of how a head had been fully severed at the neck from fence wire hit at high speed off the back of a motorbike. Or the degree of blood and tissue splattered from the man whose long hair dragged him into the lathe at high speed, wrapping him round the chuck, severing his limbs and exploding his torso in a random fashion before the machine abruptly stopped to leave an unrecognisable mass of blood, bone, clothing and oil. The reality creates a question; is man built and designed to deal with such devastation? I'm fairly certain God put me on this earth to harmonise, help and love my fellow humans. That I do to the best of my ability. But sometimes...... just sometimes, dealing with a poor soul, lost in his own emotion and despair who has taken his own life in a particularly grisly fashion, doesn't fit my criteria. He hasn't allowed me to help him, to love him, and give him the compassion and sympathy he deserves. Leaving me with a body deceased for long enough to allow nature to attempt to take it back. And a sight and smell memory to add to my bucket.

CHAPTER 25. A CLASH OF HEADS.

There are times when being near to a serious case had a different outcome. Kingstanding is a bustling and thriving suburb in the north of Birmingham. It's a mixed area of both social and private housing but is busy, and at its heart is a roundabout, known as 'The Circle', which having six exits, provides access in all different directions, and as such was a good place to 'standby' to get speedier access; that is, park up and monitor the radio. One chilly autumn morning in 1996, whilst on standby at The Circle, a crew at Sandwell Hospital were dispatched to a five year old child with a head injury from a playground incident. The school was some 15 minutes at speed for the ambulance but conversely, I estimated I could make on the motorbike in about three. Playground head injuries are common and mainly benign, and I considered giving it a miss, but hadn't done a job for a while so called in and set off with only the details that a young boy had clashed with another in the playground, and had a bump to the head. A seemingly minor event that occurs in infants schools every day with little more than a few tears and needing only some TLC from a teacher or playground assistant. But this job has taught me, like I've stated before, that 'assumption is the mother of all fuck ups', and that it always pays to keep an open mind. With this I rolled into the school driveway to be met by a frantic lady who nearly pulled me off the bike before I'd come to a complete stand still. She was clearly panic stricken and crying.

"Come quickly" she blurted, "come on, he's in the office".

"OK, don't worry," I retorted. "Try to keep calm so you can show me where he is."

I tried to sound reassuring, but it wasn't working. I didn't know who this woman was, and it wasn't important, but she struck me as someone who loved and cared for the children. The bike's side-stand went down, I climbed off and removed my helmet, placing it on the tank before unclipping the pannier with all my gear in and attempting to follow the distressed lady, who by now was standing holding an open door some four or five metres away, and beckoning me frantically to hurry up. One thing paramedics try not to do is run. It is unsafe, that's true, but the real reason is that we don't want to be in a state of breathlessness to treat the patient. There is a need to maintain the ability to treat efficiently, something which is very hard to do when you're gasping and panting yourself. Often in the case of emergencies, the callers see things as such, but attending clinicians can be quick to realise that the situation is not as urgent as was thought and more often than not, the patient is not seriously ill or injured. However, the demeanour of the greeting, panicking lady didn't bode well, and I had a gut feeling that wasn't good. As I neared the open office door in front of me, a haze of panic fell silent when I entered. And often in cases of a serious nature, people on scene step back from the patient when someone shouts that the ambulance has arrived, even though it might still be a minute or two before we actually get to them.

I stood at the doorway to the secretary's office. It was quite small with the statutory big wooden desk and filing cabinets taking up a large amount of space. The lady that met me was standing next to another lady, and beyond them was a smartly dressed but somewhat dishevelled man in a suit, who I'd assumed was the head master. Their faces painted a picture of horror, and the briefest of glimpses said that they'd have given anything not to be in this predicament at this time. They looked at me as I entered, with desperation, and probably hope, but I never saw it. On the floor in front of the desk was a young boy lying on his back, who'd I'd guessed was about five years old. He wore a red collared polo type shirt with distinctive colouring pen marks splattered on the front. I'd imagined him just a short time ago seated at a noisy low desk with his classmates, with paper and plastic scissors, and glue pots and crayons in front of him, blissfully unaware of what fate lay in store. Now, he lay almost motionless, just the quiver of a hand, or a facial nerve, his mouth full of pink fluid which had spilled and spewed out to litter the carpet that surrounded his head. His eyes lay half open in only the way they do when unconsciousness has taken over. Pallor was creeping in over the colour of his face and his lips contrasted blue against the pink vomit.

I started with the briefest of questions as I leapt forward to get him onto his side and clear his airway. I knew he'd banged his head so supported it as I rolled him to keep his head and neck in line.

"Just give me a real quick idea of what's gone on. And keep it brief", I barked, like the policeman telling the naughty child off. I sensed the intellect that surrounded me and knew that with less emotional attachment than a mother would have, that the answer I would get would be succinct.

"Well, erm, Daniel was outside in the playground and came running over to Mrs Forsythe crying and saying he'd banged heads with another boy in...in...in...what I think was just a simple playground accident." Said the male figure with an uncertain tone to his voice.

One thing about working solo, is that you develop the ability to make the best use of available resources. In this case my hands were full and I needed back up, and I needed it yesterday. I turned to the lady standing nearest to the telephone. I tried to appear calm using the 'swan syndrome'. Appearing calm and collected on the outside but under the water, my feet were going ten to the dozen. I am, after all, only human.

"Can you dial 999 and hold the phone to my ear? " This time I tried to be a little calmer and quieter in my voice so as not to confuse and cause her to get flustered. She turned and picked up the phone on the desk. I started using a suctioning device inside Daniel's mouth, then continued talking in the direction of the man.

"So then what happened?"

He had a mesmerised look about him. Surreal yet still focused on his task.
"We'll.....erm....then Mrs Forsythe brought him into the secretary's office because I think she was concerned. She said over a period of minutes, that Daniel became drowsy. Errr......the first I heard about it was Clare, my secretary, calling me into her office where Daniel appeared very sleepy and wouldn't wake. Will....errr, will he errr, he be alright?"

I ignored answering the question but they already knew. The emergency operator's monotone voice rang out,

"Emergency which service please?"

"Can you put me through to the ambulance service please? This is an operational paramedic."

And upon hearing the familiar voice of one of the ambulance control girls, I summed up my requirements,

"Hazel, it's Dave on Zulu 5. Listen, can you get through to the crew coming to my job at the school and tell them I've a five year old boy in respiratory arrest following a head injury......."

My conversation tailed off. I'd told them enough of a sitrep and

I'd too much to do with limited resources. The conversation was finished off by Clare, who then promptly replaced the receiver and looked at me as if expecting another task. I was so glad that these people were there. They probably never knew just how helpful they were.

Having established he wasn't breathing, I'd already started ventilating the child, breathing for him, with a bag valve mask. This is a silicone bag, connected to a pure oxygen supply, that enabled me to push air into the boys lungs. I'd also established him to be completely unresponsive but to have a slow, bounding pulse. There was so much to do clinically; check this, do that, get intravenous access. But providing air into this poor boys lungs was so vital that everything else at that stage paled into insignificance, and would have to wait until the ambulance crew got there. My kit was beginning to become strewn over the office floor, as I knelt in the sweet smelling pink vomit, which now adorned the knees of my leathers. I continued to ventilate, check, feel and listen. Looking in his eyes, I noted Daniel's pupils to be unequal with one significantly bigger than the other. The history of a rapid decline following a bang to the head, and now this latest sign signalled a bleed in the brain. And cessation of breathing in these cases, I knew, to not be good.

Then, in a somewhat ironic way, came music to my ears, when a female voice shouted.

"Here's the ambulance!"

Until you've worked alone, under these conditions, with patients this sick, particularly children, you will have little appreciation of how relieved one can get at the opportunity of having two more ambo guys turn up in a vehicle that you know will get you out of this circumstance and away to hospital where this poor lad needed to be. This is where my earlier sitrep now came in really handy, because the attending crew already knew the severity of the case and the circumstances, and a quick visual by blokes with some experience, as Foxy and Clive were, meant I barely needed to say anything to bring them up to speed. They approached with the stretcher and before I knew it, we were en route to the hospital that this crew had just come from. I sure as hell hoped that Clive would get us there quickly.

We left only with the boy. Any of the members of school staff would have been subjected to unnecessary distress and would have got in the way. Room in the back of the ambulance was already at a premium with both Foxy and myself in there frantically trying to do the work of a whole resuscitation team between the two of us. And were we glad that Daniel's mother wasn't with us too. Working under these difficult circumstances, trying to achieve what seems like the near impossible, in the back of a moving, rocking, speeding ambulance is hard enough; but with an understandably emotional mother seeing her baby boy fade away? Nah, we didn't want to go there.

And fading he was; a sick child's pulse rate generally rises. And as they become sicker it continues to rise. Then at the point of being very sick and pre terminal the rate drops. And drops. And drops. Daniels pulse rate was already slow, but was now dropping further still. We were losing him. Half way to hospital his rate was not consistent to sustain giving his body the blood flow and oxygen it so desperately needed, and we started performing cardiac massage as well as respiratory ventilation. The hospital had already been informed of our arrival as we left the scene. Now, Clive radioed through with the grim news that we had started CPR and that our expected time of arrival was about five minutes. At this point Clive expertly reduced our speed slightly so we weren't thrown about in the back quite so much, and could perform CPR more efficiently. I don't remember what route we took, or what cars we passed, but those we did would be going about their business as usual, visiting friends, shopping or dropping the car to the garage. It was ok for them. But one mother was to get the phone call that no one should.

Slowing for the corners, with shouts of "LEFT HANDER", or "RIGHT TURN", so we could brace ourselves, then speeding for the straights, Clive got us to the casualty department, and as the sirens silenced for the last time on this journey, he shouted through to the back of the truck, "WE'VE ARRIVED!" This part of the trip is always somewhat of a relief, but my work was not yet finished. The resuscitation team were waiting outside the doors and as the ambulance reversed up to them, they were opened momentarily before we'd stopped. As we offloaded the patient I started to explain to the Accident and Emergency consultant, what had happened as we rushed the poor boy into the building. The staff rallied round with needles, drips, wires and bags of fluid. Finally off the stretcher, I completed my verbal handover but I doubted anyone was paying much attention. The pace and atmosphere of an in-hospital paediatric resuscitation is full on. Everyone has a job, and there's a job for everyone; someone at the head end, usually an anaesthetist, sorting the airway, another at the chest performing compressions, one on each arm gaining further intravenous access, taking bloods and administering drugs, then the doctor standing at the foot end overseeing, advising and running the show, and someone diarising drug regimes and management. Perhaps now it can be realised how difficult it is to manage a pre-hospital cardiac arrest on one's own, or with only two in the rear of an ambulance.

Foxy, Clive and myself retreated in silence. I breathed a selfish sigh of relief to have handed over the responsibility. But I knew it was hopeless. In times like these, as human as I am, I try not to dwell on the job beyond my performance and self critique. It doesn't pay to think of the emotional aspect, particularly of this case being a child. I completed my handover and Foxy and myself got together to fill in our paperwork, as was customary in all patients brought into hospital.

The guys gave me a lift back to the school to collect my bike and the mood in the returning ambulance was sombre. Children who cardiac arrest do not fare well. Their mortality is high as they don't tolerate lacking essential oxygen to their cells. We had written Daniel off. He was doomed and we knew it. Even with years of experience, dealing with death, especially that of a child, is not a nice experience, and here we were, driving away from the delivery of a boy destined to become one of God's angels. I asked myself if there was more I could have done. I reeled at having missed this detail, or that issue. But they were relative insignificancies. The facts remained; I'd got there within three minutes of the call, I'd cleared his airway, ventilated him with oxygen and performed chest compressions when his heart had failed. So if he died, I asked myself if that was a success or a failure. I decided I didn't know and concluded that......if your time is up, it's up.

Three weeks later, I received a phone call on station.

"Hey Dave, it's Foxy. You know my missus works at the hospital, well she came across the name Daniel Beechdale yesterday. She knew about that arrest we had the other week, because Daniel's sister and my little girl go swimming together, and Jane was really upset when I told her. Well, you'll never in the world guess that when she checked, it's only the same boy. He's alive! I couldn't believe it."

And neither could I. It was a blessing; impossible, improbable. But I still didn't know what sort of condition he was in. The chances are that brain damage would have set in, from the head injury itself, let alone the cardiac arrest. But I had to find out. Later on that afternoon I rode to the hospital and asked the girls on reception which ward he was on. To my surprise he wasn't on ITU as I'd expected but on a normal ward. Stopping by at the shop on my way up to the ward, I bought a teddy bear to leave with the ward staff for him if it was appropriate, and upon arriving at ward four I headed for the nurses station, and for the nearest uniformed person I could find.

"Hi, erm a bit out of the usual I know, but have you got a Daniel Beechdale here, and ……..well," I didn't know how to phrase the next request. "How's he doing?" I asked with a real air of fear for the answer.

The pretty young female nurse smiled at me with an air of, almost achievement. As she started to speak, her face pointed to what I assumed was the direction of Daniel's bed.

"Oh he's doing brilliantly. Some of his speech is coming back now but he still can't walk. We're so proud of him." Her body language emulated compassion and love for this little boy. I smiled. This was one of the relatively rare times I have followed up a case, and what a result. The nurse looked at my leathers and paramedic markings, then continued.

"Are you the paramedic that went out to him at the school? I know his mother will want to speak to you",

I became hesitant with an air of unease. I hadn't come here for this and wanted out.

"Yeah, errr yeah I was one of them, but there were others. If you don't mind I'd rather not see his mum. You've already made my day telling me how he's doing. Can you give him this?"

I reached out and handed her the teddy bear. She nodded and said she would, as I turned and headed for the door, and the lift. I'd walked about a dozen paces when I heard running footsteps approaching me from behind.

"Excuse me", came a woman's voice with a broad Birmingham accent. "Were you the bike paramedic that came to Danny?"

I don't do this job for the thanks. I do it for what I get out of it. And when successes like this happen, I've done it in the hope that this boy will be given another chance. Another chance to kick a football, use a catapult, stroke a kitten, open presents on Christmas morning, become a teenager and grow into a man. And most ambulance staff are the same, having a great sense of modesty. We don't want the limelight. That's for the overpaid footballers and filmstars. My awkwardness returned. What should I say? Deny being there or accept what I knew was coming?

With an almost shy expression, I hesitated.

"Urm.......yeah."

I desperately tried to think of what to say next. Should I apologise that he has brain damage? Was there something I'd missed? Perhaps she thought I'd screwed up somehow. But I didn't get the chance. My last word to her hadn't left my lips before she launched at me, arms flung wide open encircling my neck, and pulling me into her with some force. Her cheek made firm contact with mine and the sobbing started, getting louder and louder, interspersed with words I couldn't understand. It was like meeting a long lost cousin that had disappeared in the jungles of Borneo for a decade, then been found miraculously and brought back to civilisation. I found myself holding her with a very strange feeling of not knowing this woman, but having a tremendous sense of compassion for her; immense gratitude that her boy, her baby was still alive. As much as I have never considered myself above or more special than anybody or any other profession, here was this woman's knight in shining armour, and the person who reversed fate's attempt at taking away the very centre of her universe. The one who'd given her back something so precious, it couldn't have a value. She'd gained the result that she would have given up every single item in this world for. I didn't know it then, but he would go on to make virtually a full recovery. And I contributed to that. There can be no feeling, absolutely no other feeling like the one where you have saved someone's life and given them a second chance. Stepping aside of modesty for a moment, it was me that saved him; me that cleared his airway; me that performed CPR on him, me that cannulated him, and me that gave him drugs. And it felt so bloody good.

We remained locked together, alone in the corridor, for what seemed like ages. A couple of people had walked past and as I looked up, they looked at me and smiled as they continued on. The woman was completely oblivious to anyone else around, and I'd reached the point where embarrassment had set in. Her sobbing subsided and she stepped back, now with the embarrassment on her face, but I didn't think she cared.

"I don't know where to begin to say thanks", she started, "but, well……thank you so much. Danny's doing so well. He's got a long way to go….but……he's doing well." She paused before continuing, and I felt compelled not to leave at that point. It almost seemed like part of her therapy to let her have her five minutes. She tugged on my arm in the direction of the bed from where she had come from to reach me. Seeing this lady hadn't been something which had floated my boat, and I'd carried on with it more for her benefit than mine. But seeing Danny was definitely something I wanted; it would confirm this miracle, and a miracle it was. The biggest majority of children who have a cardiac arrest in the pre hospital setting don't survive. But this one did. I looked at Danny's bed. From the entrance to the ward I was struck with a scene from a Disney movie. Helium balloons on straight strings and soft toys by the dozen adorned the bed. So much so, that I couldn't actually see him until I was quite close. And as I stepped into view a pair of young eyes met me. I wasn't sure what I was expecting him to look like, but whatever it was, I was still a little shocked. His hair was very short and had obviously been shaved, and he'd got a huge stapled wound running above his left ear. I was looking for a smile, but I didn't get one, and his eyes had a fear in them which put me back. I guess I was subconsciously thinking he would recognise me, which was bloody stupid! This little boy had never seen me, and had probably had numerous strangers over the last few weeks give him pain and discomfort from needles, pills and potions, pulling him this way and that, and forcing him to do things which hurt. No surprise really then that he was viewing me with suspicion.

Daniel had suffered a severe head injury. A simple clash of heads in the playground with another boy had set off a chain reaction; a small blood vessel in his brain ruptured from the impact, and started to bleed. His brain is soft and his skull hard, and as the bleeding continued, pressure started to build, pushing on the parts of his brain that controlled his breathing, and as vital oxygen became deprived to his body, his brain swelled increasing the pressure further still, and providing a vicious circle which slowed breathing further still until everything started to give up. Death reached out for him, but he was out of reach, for he had allies; his teachers, me, Fozzy and Clive, the hospital emergency department staff, his neuro surgeon, the paediatric intensivists and now the nurses on his ward.

Without wanting to overwhelm Danny, following my introduction, I left. But not before his mother, Julie, gave me her contact details, asking me to keep in touch. Paramedics rarely, if ever, keep in touch with patients, but somehow this seemed right. I'm human, and I wanted to see this little boys progress. I visited him several times in hospital, each time seeing more progress. He left hospital a few months later and was launched into mini stardom in his local area. I received an invite to his welcome home party. The press got involved and Danny came to the ambulance station for a visit and a photo shoot. The two of us appeared in his dad's works magazine in the article about 'the miracle boy'. And what a miracle it had been. His health went from strength to strength and I kept in touch with the family for years, and saw this boy grow into a teenager, and a young man. I lost touch, as we so often do, but at this time of writing, I've remade contact through Facebook. Danny is still doing well; very well.

My opening words of this 'book' described the 'butterfly effect'; the series of events which happen leading to a particular pathway or bigger event. I often think that had I been further away, off sick, or just not paying attention to my radio, would there have been the same outcome? I think it unlikely. Danny was snatched back from the Grim Reaper. His work on earth isn't finished yet. God has something for him to do. Like I say, if your time is up it's up. And when it's not your turn, well, it's not your turn.

CHAPTER 26. SANTA JUST MIGHT NOT VISIT THIS YEAR.....

In determining the content for each chapter, baring in mind all the events actually happened, occasionally I like to drop on an unusual story. I mean, a lot of the chapters as interesting as they might be, are very ambo 'bread and butter'. There isn't an operational paramedic who doesn't go out to similarly described cases several times a year. But sometimes, perhaps somewhat infrequently, a job comes along, that one couldn't invent; so preposterous, its intrigue defies logic.

1998 saw the end of an era for me with the motorcycle unit, as we parted full time company. At the time, each rider generally completed a two year secondment, with a review to potentially extend for another two years. And at the completion of two fantastic tours, my then boss, Chris Jones, decided it was time for me to move on, experience new fields and develop in other areas. I, of course, at the age of 32, disagreed. The bad news didn't come as a letter, or a formal interview, but rather as a flippant remark in the corridor as we passed each other one morning. We exchanged 'good mornings', as we walked in opposing directions, and having gone several paces on, Chris stopped, turned behind me, and piped up as I headed into the garage and towards the bike unit lockers.

"Oh Bradders, by the way, ummmm, as of Monday, you're

off the unit mate. Pop into the office when you've a second and pick up your new epaulettes. You've been promoted. Well done."

He turned back and carried on walking, disappearing round the corner. I was speechless. Did I hear him correctly? I'm off the bikes? Finished? I stood for a moment. I wasn't sure which hurt the most; the decision to end my secondment to the motorcycle unit, or the fact that there had been no consultation. This was the first I was aware of any changes, and now I was pissed off for allowing Chris to walk out of view, and away from me. I needed to discuss the point, so after what seemed like an age, I hurried in the boss's direction. But it was too late. As I ran out of the other door to the rear of Henrietta Street, his car drove out of sight with a puff of exhaust fumes. My first thought on pondering, was that he must have thought he'd gotten off pretty lightly, just coming out with a statement like he did without receiving any argument against it. He knew how passionate I was about the bike unit. And to make matters worse, there had been no advertising, and no one to replace me. I was annoyed and frustrated that I hadn't been allowed to be part of the decision or to put my point across to him at the time.

Inevitably, the rest of the day became as badly memorable as the start; it rained and there were no jobs of note. I spent the day thinking of what might have been. To top it all, this being Friday meant I was now off over the weekend, with no time to argue my case or change the decision. As angry as I was, I had to accept my fate, and realise that my time doing the single best job in the whole world was now at an end. I rode back to station with a surreal head. All the memorable cases; the death, destruction, people, events and experiences whizzing around inside my brain. Frustration and acceptance had become the order, as I counted down the miles towards my return as being my last. No more would I ride along High

Street, Aston, Newtown Row, New John Street West, Summer Lane and finally William Street North. I pulled into the back of Henrietta Street Ambulance Station and parked up on the wash bay, sitting for a few moments with helmet still on and bowed slightly. The characteristic sound of BMW's flat twin engine purred beneath me. It had seen what I'd seen, been thrashed hard time and time again and cosseted with polish and love at the end of each shift. Like the ever faithful hound, it was always there for me; reliable, trustworthy and obedient. Never once had it had a days sick leave, and never once had it ever said it couldn't be bothered. A tear formed. I breathed in heavily and stopped it running down my cheek. It really was the end.

With a depressive stance, I cleaned my bike for the last time, spending a bit more time on my old faithful friend. She'd seen me well, and I doubted anyone else would love and care for her as I had done. I wheeled her into the garage, and after changing out of my wet, heavy leathers I ambled in to the office, and into the presence of the leading hand, Frank 'Smudger' Smith. Smudge was always cheerful, and as always greeted me with a smile. Being a wise man, he had some idea of how I was feeling, for he'd known me for a long time, and knew my passion. There would be no condescending remarks, and no piss taking. This was almost a time of mourning for my conception and my prodigy.

"Dave, the nets been cast mate, and there's nothing you can do. Chris has made his decision" Smudge said, with compassion to his voice.

"Yeah, I know", I returned. "The end of an era though for me."

"Well, in my experience, one door closes, one opens," he said, this time with his perky tone returning, as he threw a pair of Clinical Supervisor epaulettes in my direction with some words of congratulations. I liked Smudge. We all did. He's the nicest, most placid bloke on the planet. Not once in over 20 years did I ever see him get riled. But now, right at this point, I was in no mood for any form of pat-on-the-back. The one pip epaulettes lay on the table.

"Frank," I started with aggression in my tone. "They can take these" as I picked them up and tossed them across the desk, "and shove 'em up their fuckin' arse". He continued.

"Yeah yeah Bradders, that's all well and good, but now you're a Clinical Supervisor. You're also the Ground Commander at the Villa tomorrow". I looked at him. In silence. He looked at me. Also in silence, awaiting my reply.

"You're 'avin a laugh, ain't ya", I said. He looked slightly puzzled, as if his request was the most natural thing in the world after a bloke has been delivered some exceptionally bad news.

"What's the problem? You've worked at the Villa hundreds of times. It's a piece of piss. And you get to watch the whole match from the warm comfort of the commanders gallery up in the eves. It don't get any better mate I tell ya".

And so my fate was sealed. Inevitable change, promotion, and now a cancelled weekend through enforced work. I actually wondered if the whole thing was dreamed up by someone who just wanted me to work overtime at the weekend. I'd have volunteered for anything if it'd meant I could have remained on the motorcycle unit......

The December Saturday started like any other in Birmingham; cold, wet, drab and grey, and worse still, the radio promised a good crowd at Aston Villa's home soccer match with Arsenal. We always dreaded 'good crowds', which meant more people, more fighting, more alcohol, more collapses and more work with ever decreasing resources. I tried to be positive. The old adage that things always seem better after a nights sleep is often true, and I'd had overnight to ponder my position, which I knew from past experience was one I could not change. So thinking positively, I engaged with the idea of promotion.

Clinical Supervision was the first rung of junior management and carried one epaulette pip as a rank. And at 32 years old, with a wife, two young children and a mortgage, more money was never a bad thing. The post meant largely I would still work alone, just in a car instead of a bike, and I began to think of some of the benefits; windows I could wind up when it rained, a heater, a comfy seat......oh the advantages were endless. The thought of supervising did fill me with a degree of trepidation. Guys and girls I'd worked alongside for years, stood next to at the back of the casualty department drinking coffee and watching them smoke as we gossiped and chatted about nothing, would now have to be supervised, managed, and steered towards making themselves available quickly at hospital, which theoretically did not involve drinking coffee or having a fag. This would take thought and the soft approach.

Kick-off at the football match was 1500hrs, and as usual we needed all ambulance staff at the ground an hour or so before, for resourcing and briefing. I collected the MISU (Major Incident Support Unit) and together with a front line ambulance and three other qualified paramedics, we set off for Aston Villa football ground.

With a crowd expected of nearly 40000, St John Ambulance were providing a huge amount of manpower in the form of about 40 staff, who all took on different roles, from first aiders, commanders, nurses manning the first aid room and their own ground and staff commanders. They also complimented our vehicle resources with two ambulances of their own manned by two staff each. Of the four paramedics we provided, one would remain in the first aid room, one would position at the Holte End Stand, one at the North Stand, and I as ground commander would be up up in the commentary box with the doctor. Being high up under the eaves alongside the police command and radio operators, also had the advantage of endless cups of tea. I'd have a birds eye view of the match, and a panoramic view of the ground, and more importantly, it was warm, and I knew from experience, that the two paramedics on the pitch lines would freeze their nuts off. Standing still in sub zero temperatures, watching football for 90 minutes is no fun. Sitting drinking in a heated, elevated control room on the other hand.......

I assembled everyone in the first aid room for the briefing of the ambo and voluntary St John staff. Housing some 40 people in a room meant for 20 was cozy, and with the usual pre match excitement meant plenty of chatter.

"Right, listen up guys...." I started, expecting an attentive audience. The voices hushed in a wave across the room, as they all turned and looked in my direction. 40 clean professional and smart members of a voluntary squad whose mere presence allowed the game to take place. They were a proud sight. "As usual, thank you all for turning up. It's encouraging to see so many of you. We're expecting 39000 today, so we will be busy. And at half time they're laying on some entertainment. The RAF are parachuting Santa into the ground..." I was interrupted by a few childish squeals of delight from somewhere in front of me, which started the chatting off again. "Ok folks, settle down, come on settle down" I began again after waiting a few seconds for silence and directed myself at the staff. "Mick, can you remain in the first aid room?" Mick, a veteran paramedic of many years, developed furrows on his brow as his face crumpled up.

"Yer joking arn't ya? I'll miss the bloody game." Before I could say anything, Pauline, one of my Clinical Supervisor colleagues, piped up.

"You go Mick, and I'll stay in the warm thanks". And with

a satisfied smile, she finished with "don't get what you see about a bunch of over paid knobs kicking a football about in the freezing cold anyway". Then started the banter when Mick returned fire.

"Over paid?" He exclaimed. "These are professional sportsman, at the top of their tree...." But Pauline interjected.

"They're still knobs, and they're still over bloody paid........" I took hold of the developing argument.

"Yeah alright guys, just go where you will, and Neil, can you cover the North Stand if Mick comes this end to the Holte?" Neil gave me a confirmatory nod, and I handed over the briefing to the St John commander to distribute his staff to where he strategically wanted them. I worked my way through the room to join Raj, the doctor, and the two of us headed for the command and control room.

Raj was a tall, smart, but casually dressed man who'd arrived early and been given a hi visibility jacket by someone, that looked three sizes too big, which didn't do him any favours in the street cred and recognisable department! He came across as somewhat introverted and a little quiet, but I immediately warmed to him. This was a time where doctors were only just starting to work alongside paramedics, and many had a deep distrust of us which often came across as rude contempt. Not only did they not know our scope of practice, but some had little experience in the field of pre hospital care. A patient is a patient for sure, but throw in the added issues of a violent atmosphere, rain, poor light and extremely limited resources, and they'd be at the opposite end of their comfort zone, and this to many was alien. Not all doctors have the same speciality. A geriatrician would likely be out on a limb in the Emergency Department, without some considerable exposure. Raj on the other hand was an emergency consultant and had a fair degree of pre hospital experience, which wasn't easy to spot from his demeanour, and not having worked at The Villa football ground before added to his quiet approach.

Walking up the steep steps, through the 'away' crowd, the sun tried its best to shine upon us, but didn't do anything for the biting cold wind that whisked its way through the ground. The sea of red and white of the Arsenal fans was a stark contrast to the claret and blue on the other side of the pitch, and looking at some of the crowd I became aware of the aggression in some of their eyes. Football has the ability to turn the normally placid bank clerk, into a violent raging lout, intent on killing the opposition, with the game of football seemingly just something that occurs to unite the feuding fans.

Of course it's also a placid, family event for many, where mom, dad and the two kids come together to cheer on their side with excitement and joy. Painted faces, bare top halves, banners and air horns; all part of the supporting process. As are the crowd songs. Just where do all those people go to practice the chants and to get as in-tune as they do? Beats me. As we neared the tops of the steps, a lulled Arsenal chant of 'Villa Scum' could be heard, over and over, with a much louder response from the home fans singing 'your going home empty handed.' And all perfectly in sync. I returned my attention to the door in front of me and as I opened it, was hit by a glorious rush of warming and the sound of two-way radio chatter.

The control room was a long narrow affair with a table top work surface under the window that faced out over the Doug Ellis stand. Immaculately manicured grass lay at all angles, and the overall view was fulfilling. Several people looked up at us and gave a nod of acknowledgement before returning to their own little worlds. Intelligence had suggested problems between the rival fans and the Police had had their hands full just getting the away fans coaches to the ground without issue. Now they just had to keep them apart. Tradition had seen for many years that the two sides were kept part with their own

segregational fencing. So the determined had started wearing opposing fans colours just to be able to get in amongst them to start fighting. All seemed quiet for now, and Raj and myself took our seats alongside Deb, the St. John radio operator whose job it was to provide the communication link between me and the troops. Deb had clearly been there a short while as she'd already taken her coat off so she'd obviously warmed up. The half drunk coffee by her side provided more evidence.
"Hi Deb", I started. "How's things?"

"Well apart from the freezing cold and having to climb Everest to get into here, pretty good. You?"

"Yeah so so", I continued. "This is Raj". The two of them exchanged a lip movement with an uplift of the chin, which implied both were, for some reason, a little uncomfortable in the other's presence. Some St John staff think themselves as inferior because they're volunteers. And in the presence of a doctor sometimes felt very insignificant. Raj was clearly not settled and I got the impression he was hoping for a quiet match. I sat down, picked up some info from the shop floor through radio banter, and awaited kick off, whilst heading for the kettle for us two last ones in.

A nil nil first half passed by relatively without event. A few people presented to the first aid room with the usual ailments; an abdominal pain that pointed to being of gynaecological origin, that Raj popped down to assess and sent in to hospital, a fall down a couple of steps leading to a response from one of the crews out on the ground, and an intoxication who'd needed some intravenous fluids and careful monitoring. The whistle signalled half time and it started snowing, just gently, but the sleet was a sure sign of how cold it was outside. I'd asked for the crews to be rotated around so everyone could spend some time in the warm first aid room. The crowd chanting continued and everyone seemed to be in good spirits, if a little cold.

The air in the control room stirred and the television monitor in front of us picked up an aircraft high up. The parachute team were coming in, dressed as Father Christmas and a handful of elves. The tannoy outside could be heard informing the crowd and 39000 people stopped chanting and looked up, craning their necks to get a glimpse of Santa. The monitor, relayed on the huge screen outside to the crowds, showed several people falling out of an aircraft that was clearly pretty high up in the air. The main man was coming and an air of childish excitement drifted over the room. Deb broke the short pause of silence as we all watched the screen.

"I hope nothing happens to Santa," she said. "The children will be so upset." I redirected my stare to look at the side of her face. She didn't look at me but knew I was looking at her, instead continuing to scour the monitor.

"How could you think such a thing? Anyway, he's got magical powers so nothing can harm Father Christmas." We all gave a polite laugh and continued watching. The elves had left the aircraft first, followed by Santa. I'd guessed they weren't terribly high as their chutes opened pretty quickly, and down they drifted, all seemingly in the same direction.

With the control room high up in the eaves of the Doug Ellis Stand, and with a considerable portion of the roof over the top of us, I couldn't see much sky to be able to visualise the parachuting mob directly so continued to see them in coming on the monitor in front of me. Then into my direct view, came four or five parachutists. They were near enough to me to be able to instantly recognise them from their costumes, as they gracefully descended towards the middle of the pitch wearing green outfits with big wide brown buckles and pointy ears stuck to the outside of their helmets. But before they touched down Donna let out a gasp. I also suddenly became aware that Santa was too near to the roof of the Trinity Road Stand, and before I was able to realise it, he'd landed on it, some ten feet from the edge.

"You and your big bloody mouth," I blurted to Deb in a comedic fashion. But it fell on silent ears, as without the grace of the elves, Santa hit the roof with some considerable speed. He was now right opposite us, at the same level, and giving us a clear view of the events as they unfolded. His legs buckled under the speed of the impact as his body flattened out on the roof, and the parachute with all it's rope attachments followed, not on top of him, but laid out further along the roof, and nearer to the edge. It was clearly windy, and in the blink of an eye, the chute kept moving, nearer and nearer to the edge. This time I gasped and stood up. It was obvious was what coming, and Deb let out a shout. The Police commander sat next to me let forth something similar, and with my mouth still agape, in front of my eyes, the inevitable happened. The chute dragged him off the roof and he fell 80 feet onto the side lines.

I didn't stay to watch him hit the floor. It was a race between me and Raj, who'd get to the door first, as we both had the same intention. We needed to get to the patient now, and with a near capacity crowd, many of whom we'd got to get through, it wasn't going to be easy.

In situations such as these, when travelling to a job, where the details are reasonably known, comes the consideration of mechanism of injury. That is, the forces that will have been applied to the patient, and a potential of the injuries that he might have suffered. Fractures, head, chest, spinal and pelvic injury. Bleeding and an occluded airway from a lack of consciousness. All these have the potential for death which can be avoided if managed early and with efficiency. Often patients present with horrendously messy injuries, which aside of profuse arterial bleeding, often won't kill them before something usually easily manageable will; the airway. As I've covered before, inexperience in the pre hospital field, often directs the 'helper' towards the messy bits, and the patient has the potential for dying from something they shouldn't have. Which is why patient assessment has a specific order in which it is done, and as elements are assessed, they are corrected if needed, and the next part isn't checked until the previous one is sorted. It's a system of priority. What will kill the patient first?

Since the Bradford fire in the 1980s no football grounds in the Uk have boundary fences stopping fans from migrating onto the pitch, so as I approached, somewhat out of breath, I was glad the fans had stayed put. That wasn't to say there weren't plenty of people around the patient. A plethora of yellow high visibility jackets from St John Ambulance, paramedics, police officers and ground marshals. As I neared, the backs of many of these were oblivious that I and the doctor were now on scene and needed to get to the patient, who I have to admit, thought might be dead. I'd been to many 'jumpers', some from lesser heights, and few had survived. A gentle hand with a few firm 'excuse us, coming through' statements soon saw the patient in front of me. He had a degree of consciousness and was clearly in a lot of pain. First impression was that both his legs were badly fractured, but the acute angle of his left, and the position of his foot told me that a partial traumatic amputation was a very real possibility. And that would mean one thing. Blood loss. And lots of it. The broken ends of the bones had torn his parachute suit and from the tears was a great deal of blood. He was hosing out, and as his airway was patent at that point our priority was to stem the haemorrhage, get him off the floor, out of the cold, and into the first aid room where we could work on him with better lighting.

With someone applying manual pressure to his upper leg, we all worked towards fitting a cervical collar to give some spinal support. Under these circumstances, talking to the patient is paramount so I found my self drifting into this role, whilst looking at the bigger picture. We'd need an ambulance, ready to go with stretcher at the first aid room. A police escort to get the ambulance through the traffic to the hospital, and an alert message via Ambulance Comms to the hospital to expect our arrival, so they could have the necessary resources in place.

I became aware of two men that looked somewhat out of place in amongst us, who appeared to be fixated with the worst leg, and standing right by the patients side were pointing and discussing between themselves. One of them piped up. A guy in his forties wearing an expensive brown leather jacket. I'm guessing he imagined me in control as I'd been doing a bit of direction and phoning. He came nearer to me.

"Are you in charge? He asked rhetorically. "I'm a doctor". He'd got a tone about him that I immediately disliked, but this wasn't the arena for that. Help was help, and we might have needed him. He continued, "I'm a vascular surgeon, and my friend here is an orthopaedic surgeon."

"Well thanks gents, we appreciate your offer," I replied, but we have an Accident and Emergency consultant with us," pointing in Raj's direction. "But if we need anything more we'll....." He cut me off, as he turned to Raj, who wearing an ambulance hi visibility jacket obviously hadn't been identifiable. He stated in a loud voice.

"Well, if you're the doctor, this man's bleeding heavily and I need to look at the wound, and quickly or he'll die". First rule of thumb with the seriously injured; don't tell them they might die. It doesn't do a lot for their confidence. Clearly this doctor from the crowd hadn't much experience in the acute field with a patient who wasn't anaesthetised. Raj ignored the comment, which was followed by an obviously pissed off vascular surgeon. He started again. "Look, I don't know if you heard me correctly but........" Raj wasn't listening, but continued with his task in hand. Amongst the commotion we managed to get the patient collared, strapped to an orthopaedic scoop stretcher and lifted onto the waiting stretcher which was gently and rapidly moved towards the tunnel and first aid room. This meant going across the pitch. I walked alongside the group planning ahead. Which meant my focus was away from the direct patient management for a minute. The crowd cheered and clapped, united totally in a thanking effort for the management of the horrific sight they had all endured. I looked up. All eyes were on us and everyone was clapping. No louts, no aggression, just a united crowd. A tinge of embarrassment quickly faded as the stretcher entered the tunnel and was pushed up the slope. I ran in front and managed to get in the first aid room where a space had been cleared ready for us.

This was merely a time for us to stabilise the guy and we probably didn't have much time, so as the stretcher came to a halt, I grabbed a pair of tuff cut scissors and started cutting up each leg to remove the suit, in a sort of standard practice 'let the dog see the rabbit' manoeuvre. What I hadn't banked on, was that our man was wearing a duck down one piece suit, and as I cut each leg of it, the feathers were let loose. They were everywhere, floating all over everyone and the room. Then much of them mixed with the blood that was still being lost at a worrying amount, and stuck to us all. The whole scene resembled some bizarre tarring and feathering ritual, more reminiscent of a stag party than a medical emergency. As the leg covering was moved the full extent of the left leg injury became apparent. It had been virtually amputated in the fall, and shattered beyond hope. Fragments of bone, large pieces of muscle tissue and severed blood vessels, all mixed with a large helping of fresh and congealing blood, came together to produce a horrendous wound. Our surgeon friend reappeared, still with his same tone and mannerism, but as he caught site of the wound, he looked Raj in the eye and quickly stumped up.

"What the hell are you people doing? This man needs to be in hospital." Which was precisely what we were working our balls off to achieve. Strange that. Raj gently grabbed his arm and pulled him in near, so the sides of their faces were very close.

"I too am a consultant mate, and I'll do a deal with you. I won't enter your theatre and tell you what to do, and similarly, you fuck off out of my view and let me save this patient." Choice words. We never saw him again.

Now we had another problem. A windlass was applied to the leg to stem the bleeding and the scissors continued on their upwards journey. But at the chest, the parachute harness was still in situ, and consisted of thick steel cables that my scissors wouldn't touch. I fiddled with the clasp, but it was no good. They're obviously designed not to come off in a hurry, and especially for this paramedic who hadn't a clue how to undo it. I quickly gave up and word was sent to one of the elves to come and assist. They were only outside of the door and in a jiffy, some bloke with a wide brown belt and big gold buckle had undone the harness allowing us to remove it completely. Intramuscular pain relief had now been given and the patient was settling with a reduced conscious level. So while Raj stayed at the patients head end, looking after the airway, myself and Pauline cannulated each arm with a large bore cannula, to be able to start running some fluids into the patient and give him some better pain relief. His base line observations of pulse rate, respiratory rate and blood pressure had demonstrated that he was compensating for his blood loss, but it was important for him not to receive too much fluid which would have blown out any forming clots in his leg, so this was carefully controlled. And with his suit off we now had a better idea of the full extent of his injuries. With his bleeding controlled he was covered with blankets and loaded onto the waiting ambulance, and whisked away under a police escort. As the match was to continue, and delayed by only 15 minutes of the starting of the second half, Raj stayed at the Villa ground, and I travelled along with Neil, an ambulance technician, leaving two paramedics and the doctor for the 40000 strong crowd.

The police had arranged a motorcycle out rider escort, which has to be the ultimate in adrenaline and excitement for the driver of an ambulance. To see the bikes block every single side road, traffic island, and junction allowing the ambulance to effectively continue at a steady speed without having to slow down much, is incredible and allows safe and rapid passage to the definitive place of care, which has to be good for the patient outcome. One after the other, they block a side road preventing cars from coming out of it, then as the ambulance passes, they have to accelerate to get past the ambulance and to the front of the pack to block the next road, and so it goes on. In the rear of the vehicle I didn't get to see much of this with a total focus on the patient, and just an occasional head up to look to see where we were and to estimate how long it would be before arrival at hospital, noticing the scream of a bike engine roar past us at some un godly speed. Aston Villa's ground is approximately six miles from what was then Dudley Road hospital, Winson Green and the journey probably took us no more than 10 minutes. I lost track of time through concentration, and before I realised it, we'd arrived and the back doors were being opened by the receiving team.

Tidying up the rear of the truck following most jobs is a simple affair, and over in a matter of minutes. This one was somewhat different. Clearing up meant stopping by at Henrietta Street, and literally hosing it out with the jet wash. Such was the amount of blood that lay congealed on the floor, walls and ceiling. There were smears on every surface, every handle, every cupboard. And the feathers. Those bloody feathers. Most of us were still pulling blood stained ones from our pockets several months later. Parked on the wash at the back of the station, we aimed for a slope so the water would run out of the open back doors. And run it did; a river of abattoir crimson worked its way across the floor, feeling it's way down the slope, falling off the steps, and splashing onto the ground, before finally dropping into the drain. There aren't many jobs that require this degree of cleaning, which gives the reader an idea of the amount of blood and snot that we had to deal with.

As for Santa? His leg was surgically amputated. On the plus side though, he ended up marrying the nurse who led him back to health. And rest assured however, that the children that year didn't go without. Injured Santa or not, his magical powers still managed to get the toys to the little ones that year.

CHAPTER 27. COPING WITH THE UNEXPECTED.

In relation to what we'd gotten away with in the 80's, prank wise, the ambulance service had moved on. Many of the overt jokes were gone, and seen as bullying, racist and just plain unacceptable. Pranks now had to be covert, and victims well chosen to avoid disciplinary action. The classic one was playing a prank on someone but signing another persons name on it so the perpetrator was never known, and neither the victim or the alleged player of the act were any the wiser. This often took skill and planning and few were good at it, but some were. I'd been on the end of others blags a few times in the earlier days but never reciprocated as I didn't like it done to me, and some of the tricks were, well, over the top shall we say.

While I was still on out patients serving the clinic runs and before moving up to front line, one of the blokes whose girlfriend worked with one of the senior officers, told me that she'd told him that I'd being accused of some horrendous work crime, but didn't say what, only that I was to attend a disciplinary meeting in full uniform at 0700 on Monday at Henrietta Street Station. I was still very green behind the ear, and immediately shat myself wondering what it was that I'd done. I've always hated being in trouble and have always avoided it, keeping my nose clean and trying to be, where possible, pedantic with my work ethic. I believed him, and for days, lost sleep. Of course, come Monday I turned up in my best pressed uniform complete with tunic and peaked cap, only to be laughed at by the few in on the joke. Initial annoyance was replaced by relief, but the joke had just been plain nasty and not funny to me. I didn't see its humorous side that they did, and I still can't believe I fell for it, with no written request from management, and only the word of a colleague. How stupid was I?

Post 2000, the mentoring of trainee paramedics continued and I found myself enjoying this stage of my career as it gave me a break from the classroom teaching. It is quite a skill to stand back and let a staff member loose on a patient only stepping in when necessary, letting them go forward enough to learn and gain by their partial or horrendous inadequacies. The stepping in was always the hard bit. Not too late so as the patient suffers as a result, but not so early that the trainee doesn't get the chance to demonstrate technique. As with all walks in mentoring, some needed more hand holding than others.

One guy that didn't need much hand holding from the start, and who became a good friend was Roon Parker or Roo as he was known. Roo joined the ambulance service in the mid 90's and found himself progressing onto becoming a paramedic, from that of a technician around the early naughties, a few years after I'd started as a tutor. Roo was an intelligent guy, really friendly and with a wicked sense of humour. When it came to pranks he was a top shelf player, and carried out many that had others signature on it and never admitted to being the author but we knew. They were well played, never nasty but always funny.

Fresh out of his hospital secondment and still very nervous, I mentored Roo on one occasion with Marty Follows, another trainee who became a very good friend. The three of us were dispatched to an elderly lady with some abdominal pain and Roo was attending. His patient assessment was good and the patient was chaired from the house to the waiting ambulance where she was placed on the stretcher. Roo decided that an intravenous cannula, although not vital, was appropriate to be inserted into the lady's dorsum of her right hand. Roo's demeanour was one of complete nervousness, as this was his first real cannula placement and all humour and silliness that he always displayed was now gone. His look to me said it all; could I do this for him while he watched? Not a chance and I gently guided him towards performing the task.

"Ok, Roo set this up, inform your patient, get consent, choose and prepare the proposed point of entry and I'll hand you the gear." I said to him. He took a deep breath.

"………right. Ok. Where should I put it?" He said, his voice wobbling. In a quite hushed tone, I moved nearer to him,

"Come on Roo, you've got this mate, it's all yours."

At the time we were using Venflon cannulas. These were in varying sizes of the smallest being a 20 gauge and having a pink cap and being about 1mm in needle diameter, up to the largest, a 14 gauge having a brown cap and being about 2 to 3mm in diameter and used predominantly for the giving of copious amounts of fluids for very sick patients of this one was not. The coloured caps were removable. I asked Roo what size of cannula did he want and thought would be appropriate. Having applied a venous tourniquet to engorge her hand veins and make them stand out he looked, pondered then said,

"Errrr pink? 20 gauge? Is that right?" He asked

I looked at her hand too. Despite being elderly and under weight her veins were pretty decent and I felt that the 'standard' 18 gauge size was more appropriate, but felt that would deter Roo's confidence if he tried cannulating with it. So I took out both an 18 and a 20 gauge cannula and swapped the caps handing him the bigger bore one. He took the cannula and before I could blink, had inserted it like a pro. It was in, and it was patent. He flushed it, dressed it and on we moved without a word, him clearly feeling proud of his achievement. Following the handover of the patient to the hospital, we had a quick debrief and discussed all elements of the case in a rather routine fashion.

"How did you think the cannulation went Roo?" I asked. He replied

"Yeah, not too bad, but bugger me those 20 gauge cannulas are bigger than I remember ain't they?"

I handed him the 20 gauge cannula now with the green, 18 gauge cap, and he pondered it for several seconds before it dawned on him that the caps had been swapped. He paused, then still looking at the cannula spoke up.

"You bastard! You swapped them". His grin started and grew. We laughed, but I realised I'd woken the sleeping giant, whose motto was 'revenge is a dish best served cold'.

Each paramedic at the time had their own kit bag. They were teal blue and carried all the Gucci gear and drugs we used at the time and were designed in such a fashion that the opening of the front pocket revealed an intubation 'roll' that would literally roll out like a small picnic blanket, displaying an easy access to all the necessary gear for providing advanced airway management to a patient in a life threatening hurry such as a cardiac arrest. The gaining of these bags was a proud moment and the green beret of being a 'para'. They were the responsibility of the individual paramedic and were kept on station in a common shelf of a large cupboard that all the paramedics had access to.

One drab autumn morning some weeks after the Roo episode when all thoughts of it had been forgotten, I was working on a single responder fast response car, and had the call to a cardiac arrest in a north Birmingham suburb. I weaved my way through the traffic pulling up outside the house, alighting the car, and grabbing all my kit before quickly making my way into the house. As usual there was a flurry of emotion and panic and I was led into the front downstairs room and presented with a youngish. male aged about 30 lying on his back and having that classic cardiac arrest look about him. Visually unresponsive, eyes half open, mouth open and pale to the face. A brief question to the older lady standing now above me enlightened me to him having been found in this position when she came downstairs having heard him call out before then hearing a bump, presumably of him falling. He been there about 10 minutes I figured and I proceeded to a resuscitation protocol. I set up the defibrillator next to him and where I could see it, cut off his upper clothes and applied the monitoring/defibrillator pads to his chest while turning on the machine. As is so often the case, automated actions saw me looking at the monitor but reaching to my bag to open it for all the kit I would need. A quick unzipping of the side pocket let the airway kit roll out which it did, right in front of the patient, me, and the older lady standing over me watching, now joined by several others in the room from where they came I did not know.

Along with all the airway kit now presented in front of us all, was something else, to which I had to do the double take. It was a magazine. And it fell with the front cover facing up, and in the right orientation for all the standing onlookers to see. 'Big Boobs Monthly' proudly displayed a topless lady on the front with an enormous pair of pouting breasts and a smile as big, with her hands on her hips. Just looking at us! What does one do when presented with this situation? Cardiac arrest mode does something for one that few activities do; it creates a total, unadulterated focus that little to nothing will detract, including a visual anatomical reference of the female naked body. Ironically I don't even recall thinking where it had come from. Sure, it was a surprise, but I moved it out of the way and continued with my quest.

The crew arrived and the resuscitation attempt was ceased with no hope of survival. The scene was cleared up, paperwork was completed and I left, only then having the opportunity to contemplate what had happened. I don't think that Roo had anticipated the magazine actually falling out during a resuscitation effort but that I would have spotted it upon a kit check. But kit checks were rarely done because these bags were our own and only we used them so we all knew that our own bags were good to go. It had been a classic revenge prank and one I deserved and in hindsight, knew was coming. I saw Roo some days later and recounted the tale of what had happened and how his plan had worked better than ever he could have imagined. The dish had indeed gone cold!

Marty completed his paramedic course with Dal Wade, and around the time of the enormous boobs exposure, I found myself mentoring the two of them on the road. Dal was patient caring on a doctor's urgent removal of an elderly male with abdominal pain. The nature of the case meant we approached it at normal road speeds and without the use of blue lights and sirens. We pulled up outside a main road address in Erdington and all got out, following Dal inside a small block of flats, where a set of stairs led us to the front door we sought. Dal knocked and we waited, me standing back, as by now the boys had a fair bit of experience and my input was minimal.

"I'm coming….. Hold on" was heard from inside the flat. It was the unmistakable accent of an elderly Jamaican male, and through the fire retardant glass of the front door we could see the brown clothing of a man wearing a trilby hat who opened the door.

"Hello sir" said Dal, I'm……."

But the man had already walked off back into the flat saying

"Come hin, come hin".

Now Dal was clearly an intellect, but wasn't the sharpest knife in the draw when it came to communication and common sense. We all followed the man into the lounge who now was seated on the settee not appearing to be in much if any discomfort, legs apart, sat forward and leaning on his walking stick. He was wearing a brown pin stripe suit with a mustard coloured shirt, brown tie and a dark brown trilby hat and looked very dapper, as if he was going to a wedding. Looking around the room, it was clean and tidy but so very 70's, with flowery wallpaper and yellow glass shelving with ornaments. The carpet wouldn't have looked out of place in a pub or a bingo hall, and the television was clearly old. Dal started again,

"I'm Dal. What's your name?"

"Hmmmm?" Came the reply. "What you say? Dal repeated the question.

"Speak hup!" The man came back with a short, blunt statement "I bin to me doctor dis marnin……." Dal cut him off.

"WHATS YOUR NAME?" He now shouted.

"Hmmmm? It's Leon. Ya don't need ta shout. I's not deaf"

Dal was becoming irritated and Marty and I looked at each other with a smile starting and a giggle on the horizon. Dal spoke again with a slightly lowered volume.

"WHATS THE PROBLEM LEON"

"Hmmmm? Well I gat a problem wid me stick" Leon replied. Dal had a puzzled look on his face. "WHAT DO YOU MEAN, YOUR STICK?" Leon continued.

"Me stick man, me stick. I got a problem wid me stick". Marty and I were cottoning on in which direction this was going and the giggling neared, but clearly Dal was on another planet. He continued,

"I DON'T UNDERSTAND WHAT YOU MEAN. WHAT'S THE PROBLEM WITH YOUR WALKING STICK?" Leon stood motionless for a few seconds staring at Dal. Then, despite being clearly the only person living in his flat, he leaned forward, looked left and right, then in a hushed voice spoke directly at Dal.

"We're all men togedder, let me show you….." Dal still continued to look puzzled, but I prepared for the onslaught. Leon stood upright, leaned his walking stick up against the settee, unzipped his trousers and placed his hand inside the fly opening. But it didn't stop there. His hand went further and further in to the depths of his trousers; deeper and deeper until his elbow was at the fly opening. His hand started to come back out again and like a snake handler managing a python out it came. A penis of gargantuan properties. Resembling a babies arm holding a blood orange, with a girth and length to make most eyes water. I don't recall which was funnier; the site of Leon getting his penis out or Dal's face, now looking at something so huge, and so unexpected, he was totally lost for words. He stood there, mouth open, eyes wide and completely paralysed for something to say. Probably the latter.

My professionalism, I'm afraid went straight out of the window and to save face, I grabbed the kit bag and walked quickly out of the flat and down to safety of the ambulance where my laughter could be set free. And set free it was. I have always had this issue that when I find something funny, I'll laugh until it hurts and then some. At the point that my abdominal muscles were aching so badly the boys and the patient came downstairs and just as I'd got myself together the back doors opened and in got Dal and Leon. I sat in the front passenger seat, with Marty driving, with neither of us talking and me looking out of the side window, for fear of setting off the giggles again. Dal however didn't at all see the humour even after the patient had been handed over to the staff at the hospital, when we were debriefing and discussing the matter, when of course the laughing restarted. It transpired that Leon had got retention of urine and had the associated abdominal pain, but had assumed the problem lay with his penis.

Around 1996, when I was deeply seated (pardon the pun) on the Motorcycle Unit, I received a call to a cardiac arrest in south Birmingham. It was one of those autumn days full of cloud but was light and airy. The temperature was mild and with the roads being dry, was one of the calls I loved. I'd started from the city and made good progress, weaving in and out of the traffic, sirens blazing and making short work of the roads. After about 4 or 5 miles I pulled up outside of the address, and placing the bike on its side stand, alighted, removed my helmet and unclipped the pannier, carrying it in to the patient. The dwelling was a terraced affair, situated on a main road and of the type which was either a current, or ex council house. There was a middle aged woman standing at the open front door, with her arms folded and wearing somewhat of a shabby looking, hand knitted jumper. She didn't appear to have the demeanour of panic and as I approached her she piped up.

"You don't need to rush bab, 'ers bin gone a while". Regardless of what a loved one says under these circumstances, we need to access the patient quickly to be able to decide ourselves on the timing of getting in and doing something.

Having politely asked the lady to lead me to the patient, a slight hesitation in her mannerism, saw her unfold her arms, raise her eyes, and walk inside the house, transcending the stairs, for me to follow her. The stairs moved us towards the rear of the house and from the landing, she pointed into the bathroom at the far end of the corridor. A brief pause to determine what I was seeing, pointed out what appeared to be a very small, lower part of a body hanging over and into the bath, with the top half out of view. As I approached, I could see the top half of an elderly female dangling into the bath tub with fluids, clearly having come from the lady's mouth adorning the tub and having dried. She'd been here a while and the lady who met me at the door had been correct. At least in my initial estimation. I put the motorcycle panniers down on the bathroom floor and put on a pair of barrier gloves. The patient was cold, and clearly deceased, probably having passed several hours before because she had rigor mortis present. This is a stiffening of the muscles after death which comes on after about 4 hours, lasting for several hours more before relaxing, and the body ends up stiffening in the position in which it dies. This means that for this poor old lady who'd died hanging over the bath, probably vomiting and feeling so unwell, she'd kneeled over the bath to vomit, and died in that position.

I turned to look at the lady who'd met me at the door. Her facial expression painted a picture.

"I told you so!" And all I could do was acknowledge this but accept that I had to do what I had to do. And so the formalities started, of who I was and who she was. Having decided the situation was not suspicious, I moved the deceased into the bedroom. She was a tiny, elderly lady about 4 foot nothing in height and weighing probably no more than 20kg wringing wet. The plan was to place her on the bed, which offered her more respect than hanging over the bath. I picked her up and carried her across the landing and into the bedroom, whereupon I put her on the bed. However, her rigor mortis prevailed meaning she lay on her back with her legs
sticking up in the air, bent at the knees. As was customary at the time, a sheet was placed over her, producing a mound which stuck up off the bed by the length of her upper legs. I had no choice and although it looked a little odd, I left her in this state and went downstairs.

The deceased's daughter as it turned out was a lady by the name of Julie and despite the initial impression I gained of her being less than ideal, she actually turned out to be rather a nice person. Practical and not emotional, and clearly a realist, Julie informed me that the deceased was a 90 year old who had been living on borrowed time for many years and who had a significant medical history. She offered to put the kettle on as I confirmed the process following death in a private residence that didn't involve suspicious circumstances. The Police would attend as a matter of course, acting as coroners officers, and so I updated ambulance control and awaited the arrival of others.

The sounds of the spoon stirring the tea cups was interrupted by a knock on the door from the police. In walked a WPC, clearly experienced and leading the investigation, and a young male officer who was clearly the opposite and perhaps within his first week of operational duty, or at the least, attending his first domestic death, and looking very green behind the ear. After introducing themselves, I took them upstairs to view the body and the male of the partnership was instructed to remain with the body for continuity of evidence. He settled himself in the chair within the bedroom and myself and the female police officer went back down stairs. Small talk filled the lounge room for a short while at which point I realised that I'd left something upstairs and went up to retrieve it. At the top of the stairs I was met by a frantic young policeman, running towards me, screaming!

"AAAAAAHHHHHHHHH".

He had a look of sheer terror on his face as he ran past me with such determination, that the two of us very nearly both ended up in a heap at the bottom of the stairs. I could hear what sounded like a zombie cry coming from the bedroom, and having continued on to where the deceased lay saw her final movements as she'd sat up then flopped over from the weight of her legs finally toppling her up and over, and the air in her lungs coming up and out and giving the impression of a 'moan'. It's a common sound we hear when picking up the dead off the floor, as the air in their lungs makes its way up through the vocal cords. To the young copper however, there was no clinical explanation to explain his experience aside of the living dead having come back to haunt him! He exited the front door and in a very shaken state he sat in the police car and refused to come back into the house. Julie was none the wiser of the event, but I shared it with the WPC and of course at the time, away from listening ears, we found the event hilarious. In hindsight, and with several more years under my belt I now really feel for that young bobby. For all I know it may have frightened him so much it may have scarred him for life and prematurely ended his career. I never gave it a thought to go outside to him and explain what had happened to console him and give him reassurance.

CHAPTER 28. THE FLYING CAR

One thing that paramedics experience on a regular basis, is a transition from calm to chaos in the blink of an eye. Some cope well with it, others not so. In my early days at Henrietta Street Ambulance Station, there was a bloke, Bob, who'd served about 10 years and who left to go and work at the Rover factory in Longbridge Birmingham. 20 years before had seen many do the same, reasoning better money and less night shifts. Bob on the other hand told me that he could no longer cope with not knowing what lay ahead of his working days. He needed to know exactly where he'd be at any given time on any given day, and know that at the end of his shift, he would be heading for home free from having witnessed the death of a child and not covered in shit and snot. For this reason, the prospect of working on the assembly line putting together Austin Metros and Montegos knowing that at 10 o'clock in the morning he'd be in the same place, on the track, doing the same boring and mundane thing that would be his future for the next 20 years was infinitely more attractive than manning an ambulance on 'front line'. As a young upstart I couldn't see his logic, but as time went on I got it.

Attending a serious case gives a strange post job retrospect of just what has happened, following a period of calm and rest at the station awaiting for the incident to come in. I often look back at death and think that when I had been making a cup of tea in the morning, this traumatic deceased male I'd been to was going about his business completely unaware that shortly, he'd be dead; and in a particularly gruesome way.

As part of the motorcycle unit I was often called upon to attend public relations events. The bikes were big news and always created a furore whenever we rocked up to a public gathering. One beautiful summers day around the mid 90's I was asked to attend such a gathering east of Birmingham, towards Coventry. It was a stinking hot day and towards the mid afternoon, I was looking forward to going home and getting out of my hot leathers. The day had been a relaxing one, as not technically on operational duty, I'd switched off to response knowing the radio or phone wasn't about to send me on an adrenaline fuelled ride into the unknown. I could relax, chat to the people then retreat. Which is exactly what I did. The route home would take me along the A45 into Birmingham, but with light nights, awesome sunshine and the prospect of windy lanes with little traffic, I decided to take the scenic trip back through the picturesque village of Hockley Heath. This lies on the outskirts of Birmingham and routes to Stratford. It's surrounded by fantastic roads that are a Mecca for bikers and boy racers. Traffic was light, the roads were dry and the ride home promised me plenty of smiles as I'd be putting in a *progressive* ride for educational and personal development benefit; ahem.....

I indicated left off the A45 and at the traffic roundabout, signalled left again. Few cars meant I could smoothly negotiate the turn without stopping, then into a 30mph zone in the lead up to the village. As an advanced motorcyclist, speed limits in the restricted areas are strictly adhered to when not responding to an emergency, and even then, the speed is very carefully and dynamically thought about. After all, a 30mph zone is 30 for a good reason, as is a 40mph and so on. Riding at this speed gave me chance to enjoy the cooling air after the long hot day and created a chilled ride to negotiate the built up area. At the end of the village is a lane which leads back to Birmingham and is the one I'd planned on taking. Seeing it approaching, a mirror check preceded a right turn indicator, a slowing down, then a shoulder check before tipping the bike in and making the turn. There is a short section of road here which maintains the speed limit before the national speed limit sign is reached just after the first right hand bend. The national speed limit sign is affectionately referred to in police motorcycle training as the 'GLF' sign, standing for 'Go Like.....'. Where appropriate, it is the area where most progress can be made and is the sign I was anticipating seeing and doing something with. Fate, however had other plans.....

I rounded the corner and prepared to drop a gear, but rather than accelerate, I slowed down to speak with a frantic driver coming towards me with his arm out of the window waving madly. He clearly wanted my attention. I pulled up alongside him facing in his opposite direction. The car was a small sporty hatchback and the driver was a young guy of about 20, with long hair and a grubby tee shirt. He had the remnants of an attempt at a moustache which was kind of lopsided with more hair on the one side than the other, but overall a pretty unmanly look. It complimented his acne well though and he was clearly out of breath and panicking. His waving stopped and he'd started speaking before either of us had pulled up so I didn't catch what he was saying, especially with my helmet on. I lifted the face part so I could hear him properly.

"Calm down mate and tell me what the issue is" I said. Unable to calm, he blurted out again

"Down there, about a mile mate. Hurry up I think he's dead"

Before I could ask just what was going on, he drove off. I turned my head expecting to see him perform a U turn and come back to let me follow him to whatever lay ahead. Alas no. The spotty driver did not return, leaving me wondering what was going on. His panic and demeanour clearly implied that there was something serious up ahead so I called it in to Metro Control to see if they'd had any calls for an incident in the area. They hadn't. This is one of those times that we go into an incident knowing very little of what we'd find. Was it someone shot at a house, or perhaps a hit and run road traffic accident? What dangers would present to me? I cautiously rode forwards but with progress. Now in the GLF zone, this wasn't quite the ride I'd planned and I was now back in work mode. I worked on the assumption of finding something in or on the road and it wasn't long before I could see something up ahead. It looked from a distance to be an old blanket or a bag lying still in the road. As I got closer, however, the familiar site of blood and exposed tissue painted a different story. It was a body; male by the clothing and teenage to 20's I guessed. He was very obviously deceased and had injuries incompatible with life. His legs were both severely fractured, twisted with one lying upright on his chest and the other underneath him. One of his arms was partially amputated below the elbow and part of his head was missing with exposed brain tissue visible. His face was distorted with deep scrape lines adorning the injured side. From his position, there was a trail of blood, tissue and fluid leading away from me and for some distance. I considered that this poor guy had been carried down the road possibly underneath a car. The question remained then of where was the car? Still on scene or was it the young male who'd stopped me earlier? With no other vehicles or people around I figured the car I'd seen earlier was connected to this death, but with such horrendous injuries I didn't notice any damage to the front of his vehicle which made it odd for a hit and run.

I parked the bike up in a protective position for any other approaching cars and walked towards the body where upon my suspicions were confirmed. Calling it in, I asked for police and an ambulance crew to attend and asked for Metro to standby and await a further sitrep (situational report). A look around the scene demonstrated some big gouging marks on the road which started some way back and led off the tarmac and onto the grass verge. A hole had been created in the hedge and this started to display a more logical explanation. A vehicle had gone through this hole, had created the skid marks and by the length of them had been travelling at speed.

There was nothing I could do for the deceased in the road so I followed the trail through the hole in the hedge. On the other side, the ground dropped away sharply with steep bank to sit about 4 to 5 metres lower than the road, and the terrain here was mainly thick wooded trees. The pathway of the vehicle was very visible and following it by eye from the hedge I spotted it. A small Peugeot 205GTI perched precariously but wedged in a tree about 3 metres from the ground and upright. It had sustained colossal damage with every panel looking like it had been through a crusher. The roof was pushed down and the bonnet was partially up with the whole front end caved in. A wisp of what looked like steam emanated from the front of the bonnet. Adorned up the side and covering the wheels were mud and grass, and there didn't look like there was any glass left. My next and obvious issue was whether there was anybody else either in the vehicle or ejected and lying in the woods, and from my position on the wood side of the hedge, at the top of the bank I was able to look slight down at the car which was now about 30 metres from me. In the rear seat I could see someone; clearly a person and moving.

As is the norm for being first on scene at a multi casualty event, my job was to initially ensure my safety, then using the mnemonic METHANE, I got back on the radio with my sitrep; M stands for Major incident, an indication to those in comms who need to rally resources, such as helicopters, roads crews, doctors and other such responders. E is for Exact location, T is the Type of incident, H to report on any Hazards such as fire or chemicals, A is for Access and Egress, N is for Number of casualties which at that point consisted of one deceased and another moving, but totally unknown patient, and finally E is for Emergency services present and needed. From my vantage point now still relatively high up, I could survey the area for any obvious persons involved and perhaps lying dead or injured on the floor. The normal process is to survey the scene thoroughly for numbers of casualties for this in the long term saves more lives than merely attending the first casualty that is come across. This information can then be relayed back to comms who can organise appropriate resourcing. My problem here was that the car first off was in a tree 3 metres off the ground. I knew there was one person inside but couldn't see any others from the position I was in. The car was a relatively long way from the body on the road and if others had been ejected, that would mean a large search area, in a rural, heavily wooded environment that would normally be carried out by a team of fire fighters using thermal imaging cameras to expedite the job. I was on my own, and in this isolated location didn't even have other motorists or householders to help, who when present are generally a God send to single paramedics.

I surveyed the scene but couldn't see anything obvious to indicate other casualties, and I knew I'd be alone for a while so planned to see if I could help this guy still in the car. Helmet off, I grabbed my clinical equipment from the motorcycle, stored in the rear panniers; defibrillator, oxygen, monitoring equipment, drugs, fluids and field dressings to name but others, all conveniently packed into small cases for carriage. We didn't have the room to store large quantities of equipment and I was hoping that help and with it resupply, wouldn't be too long.

One of the first elements instilled into all first responders is that of self preservation and personal safety. After all, an injured paramedic requires an extra ambulance; one for them and one for the original patient. Plus, an injured or dead paramedic can't attend to the needs of the scene injured and so in the case of a major incident, more people will die because there is one less responder. There had been a case many years before of a nurse who came across the scene of a chemical tanker involved in a collision on the motorway with chemicals gushing out all over the road. Without a thought for her own safety, she proceeded from her car to walk through the liquid to attend to the injured persons. However, the liquid was highly concentrated acid, and she literally dissolved into it and died. However, what an individual does or does not do on scene in relation to safety is highly subjective. What one considers is safe to proceed into, another may have different opinions, and as a paramedic there is often a level of danger which has to be considered, with attempts to mitigate the situation. If no responder treated any patient, or entered any scene until things were 100% safe, then nothing would ever get done. Paramedics enter unsafe scenes all the time but usually as part of a crew where each looks after the back of the other and an extra set of eyes and opinions is vital. I have laid in the back of an upturned vehicle tending to trapped patients, with petrol dripping onto me from a ruptured fuel tank. It is often not until there is retrospective consideration and reflection on the cases we deal with that a realisation of a safety issue arises by which time its over and done with and more by luck than judgement, I wasn't injured.

I had to think about how I was going to get to the patient stuck in the car that was now 3 metres up a tree. As I approached the car I could see it was severely, and what looked like securely stuck in its position wedged in amongst the heavy branches, and I estimated it wouldn't move easily if I climbed up. I knew this model of car would mean the presence of petrol, and that always heightens my senses for fire, especially where batteries and broken cables were concerned. On arrival at the car I shouted up to see if there was any response, and a panicked, breathless voice replied. I offered calming reassurance and told him things were going to be ok, and that help for him was here.

"I can't……breathe" he stated, clearly breathless, and that didn't bode well, although I'd still to climb up and examine him.

"Try to keep calm mate", I said, as I reached up for the best route to get me to him. Although we always ask the panicking to remain calm, in the face of it, that's pretty impossible to do from their perspective but I reckon just the mere presence of someone willing to help is reassurance and somewhat calming. I got level with the rear of the car and wedged myself against the tree. Peering in to the car I could see a young, late teens male sat on the back seat, the roof down towards his head making it impossible for him to sit upright. He was wedged into a small space between the roof and the seat and my only access was through the smashed rear window opening. He was relatively free of visible blood, but clearly breathless, anxious and fidgety. He again stated with concern to his voice.

"Help….me. I can't breathe",

The words being spat out quickly to enable him to get another shallow breath in.

"Give me an …….inhaler".

I asked him his name, but he didn't reply with the answer, only continuing with his plighted request for breathing relief.

In circumstances such as these, my priorities were to stem any exanguinating bleeding, of which there wasn't any visible, ensure his airway was clear, and his breathing was adequate, before moving on to assess his circulatory system. With his airway patent, a listen to his chest with a stethoscope revealed air entry to both sides but his lower lung fields were very bubbly. I discounted the presence of a tensioning pneumothorax, a severely life threatening condition that is relatively easily treated by the insertion of a long needle into the chest wall, but the sound of bubbling in his chest and the history of severe trauma, now with breathlessness meant one thing; a haemothorax - bleeding into his lungs from somewhere, filling them up and reducing his ability to breathe. This is treatable only on the surgeons table and that would be some way off. All I could do was monitor him for signs of worsening, looking for an increasing respiratory rate and a raising of the point at which bubbling could be heard in his chest. If this lad went into cardiac arrest, there was nothing I could do for him but watch him die. He was stuck in the car by encapsulation and I couldn't get access to perform CPR. I applied oxygen to him but his panicked state just kept ripping it off; not a good sign and demonstrated a worsening of his condition.

A further updated sitrep was given to Metro Control asking for the helo (helicopter) to attend. This was his only chance. Basic observations of pulse rate, respiratory rate, blood pressure measuring, oxygen saturation assessment, cardiac monitoring and neurological assessment carried out on a calm, cooperative patient laying flat and still in bed, with adequate lighting and a colleague to record findings and assist with the procedure is easy in comparison. Here was a poor lad, sat almost upright, head at an angle against the roof, panicked and anxious, totally uncooperative and in a precariously balanced car, stuck several metres up a tree with my only access to him through an open shattered window, the smell of petrol heavy in the air and just hoping that if this case went tits up I could jump off and hopefully not break my legs. At the time, my thought process was focussed entirely on being there and doing what I could. There wasn't a great deal I could do with the resources I had to hand, but monitor and hope for a speedy backup.

In these circumstances, time seems to go by very quickly and often, what seems like 10 minutes turns out to be 30. I heard sirens. At least we could now work towards a plan for this patient, and within minutes the Fire Service were parking up and setting up. The officer in charge approached me and shouted up. Normally I'd get together with him and brief him on what the situation was and what I wanted of him. But this had to be done from 3 metres up. A search of the area was initiated and more resources called for. The fire guys worked towards securing the car as best they could and cutting gear was hauled up the tree to get the roof off and give me more access. Ordinarily, spinal injuries are a major consideration in cases of trauma, but this guy was going to die of his respiratory issues way before any spinal problems and although thought about, the teams priority was to get him out.

In hindsight, I wondered what he had been thinking. Was my presence helpful to him? Just how much reassurance was I providing? One has never seen true panic until they've witnessed someone completely and utterly consumed with trying to breathe, and being unable to do so. The vicious circle meant the more increased his work of breathing became, the more oxygen his body demanded from a system that just couldn't supply it.

The Fire guys worked tirelessly like a swarm of bees, sweat dripping of them as they meticulously laboured to save this poor lad. My fears for him worsened as his agitation worsened, and he became panicky and more uncooperative - a sure sign of reducing oxygen to the brain. I'd gained intravenous access to his right arm with a large bore cannula and had fluids running to prop up his failing blood pressure. Where bleeding is occurring, the body's natural clotting process start in an attempt to stem the loss. IV fluids work to build blood pressure but it is a balancing game; push the pressure up too much only blows the clots out worsening bleeding, but where the pressure drops too much, then cerebral tissue oxygenation falls effectively killing the brain. Systolic blood pressures are maintained around 110mmhg in the case of head injuries to maintain cerebral perfusion. In the case of no head injury but where there is major bleeding, we can allow a drop to 90mmhg. Where the bleeding is compressible, that is, where we can put pressure on a wound such as a leg or arm, this assists with haemorrhage control, but this patient had bleeding into his chest cavity which I couldn't manually stop, and his lung sounds indicated they were filling further with blood. This bloke was dying, and there was nothing I could do to save him.

My body started to ache in the position I was holding myself in, wedged between the tree branch and the car, and I became aware of the sweat dripping off me. I was sticky and over heating wearing heavy protective leathers, and decided to ditch the jacket and throw it to the ground. With ropes and ladders forming a scaffolding, the fire guys reached what was left of the car and started the arduous task of removing the roof. Continuously giving reassurance and guidance to the patient of what was happening, failed to give him support. When the hydraulic cutters pierced a roofing support post, the bang would startle him, setting him back off on his quest of demanding inhalers or oxygen. As his conscious level reduced further, the roof was hinged forward to give me more access and the patient more room. But this improvement in environment wasn't the answer for him.

I'd probably been on scene for about 40 minutes when the familiar and reassuring 'chop chop chop' noise of a helicopter's rotors progressively getting louder filled the air. If anything was going to save the patient, whose name I still didn't know, it was this mode of transport. It landed in a nearby field and within minutes the slightly out of breath helo paramedic and doctor appeared. Although I dislike ever leaving the side of a patient in these circumstances, I couldn't give a proper handover from 3 metres up. So I motioned for the paramedic to join me in the tree, and climbed down to speak to the doctor, whereby both of them could hear, but hopefully the patient not so much. It's never a good thing to speak about how near death a patient is in front of them, and decorum dictates a little bit of common sense. I didn't know either of the helo boys but we worked well together, and the decision was taken to 'scoop and run' - a process of a controlled 'pulling out' of the patient from his predicament and transport him quickly. There are few occasions where speed is of the essence, but this sure was one of them. The spinal board, a long flat piece of equipment designed to keep the patient in line to help with spinal care was used to relatively quickly get him out and down on to the ground where another rapid assessment was carried out to confirm how near death this young man was, and with the help of the fire guys, he was carried the short walk to the helicopter. Only when he was out of my care was I able to breathe that huge, huge sigh of relief and somewhat relax back. Now wasn't the time for reflection. That would come later, and only between me....and me. This was before the days of debrief and group chats to determine what went well and what needed development.

Before long the sound of the air being broken by chopper blades signalled the takeoff and away to the nearest major trauma centre, at the time Selly Oak hospital, Birmingham and the medical trauma team. It was now out of my hands and into the realms of fate who would decide on this young guys life. I tidied up my equipment which at this point looked like a tornado had moved through it, decimating every crevice and stripping all the consumables. My bags went back into the motorcycle panniers somewhat lighter than they went in. It was now nearing 8 o'clock and the air was cooling slightly. I picked up my leather jacket and briefly watched on as the fire fighters also cleared up the last of their gear. We thanked each other and alighted our designated vehicles. I pushed the starter button and the bike resumed into life, but it was some time before that clutch lever was engaged and the gear was selected. I sat there in contemplation of what had gone on. We might be paramedics, but we're still human, and as much as we try not to dwell on the negativity of fate, it creeps in. I wasn't hopeful of the out come of this one.

The ride home was not what it should have been, and as the sun set over the gas towers back in the city, I pulled into my base station, now Hobmoor Road Ambulance Station in the Eastern suburb of Small Heath, Birmingham. Nobody was on station, which was all in silence. I washed the bike and put it to bed, then restocked my kit, changed my gear for my own private leathers, then mounted my own bike and rode home in the darkness. The fun of riding for the moment having been stripped from me.

Mid morning the next day, the phone rang. It was the police.

"Hey Dave, it's Dan from Stechford nick. Mate, can we get together sometime soon? I need a statement about the fatal yesterday."

I wasn't sure whether he meant the initial deceased in the road or the guy I'd worked on. Even though I knew his chances were slim...very slim, I kind of hoped.

"Did the evacuated lad make it?" I asked with hope.

"Nah mate. He was pronounced deceased upon arrival at Selly Oak. He arrested in the chopper en route."

His words were said with no feeling. No emotion. This police officer hadn't been there and was just passing on information. He was only doing his job but his conversation was just, well, emotionless. And emotionless it should have been. We're medical professionals who deal with death frequently and it doesn't pay to get involved emotionally. But we're also human, and when I work on my own there is no one to bounce the job off. No one to tell it like it was, how I felt, what I did, and what I couldn't do. Could I have done more? Should I have? The patient's death was recalled so very matter of fact by the officer on the other end of the phone, who went on to tell me that the double fatal was caused by a race between the guy in the car who stopped me and the Peugeot. Its driver had been ejected and crushed by the rolling car, and his front seat passenger, ending up in the back. Neither deceased had been wearing a seat belt. The other driver had handed himself into a police station and subsequently arrested for dangerous driving. And the two dead young guys? A pair of parents received a knock on the door that night to tell them their beloved boys had been killed by someone's stupidity and dangerous driving.

I've dealt with this scenario many times both before and after. More recently, in Australia a similar scenario of ejected persons being killed by not wearing a seat belt in a rolling car. It's not difficult to clunk click, but adrenaline and in some cases alcohol cloud the judgement. The scenario of *'it'll never happen to me'*, doesn't always come true as these poor examples demonstrate. And for me? This case and all the others might be adding add to my stress bucket. Will it ever overflow…….only time will tell.

CHAPTER 29. MOTORWAYS AND FOOTBALL DON'T MIX.

From my earliest memories of being in the Ambulance Service, one job I aspired to more than anything was the mobile incident officer, known by its call sign of Mike Oscar 1. (MO1). Only one on duty at any one time, their role was to provide officer support across the region, and came particularly into function out of hours when many station and senior officers, who only generally worked 0800 to 1600hrs, had gone off duty. They were to some degree general drivers, security staff and dogs body to the crews. If an ambulance broke down or couldn't function for some reason, MO1 would turn up and sort them out another vehicle at 2 o'clock in the morning. And if a garage door malfunctioned and the crews couldn't secure a station, it was the mobile officer who again came to keep a watchful eye on things while they were out. These mundane tasks didn't interest me at all. But what did, was their primary reason for existence; to command the scene at serious incidents.

Imagine the scene; two vehicles in a head-on collision on a dangerous section of country road. It's dark, raining and cold. There are three teenagers in one car, and four elderly people in the other. This has the potential for requiring more resources than may be available at the time, and needs some serious scene management. How many casualties are there and what are the injuries of the occupants? Do their ages demand specialised resources either to scene or to the hospital? How many ambulances are needed? Which hospitals do which patients go to? And when the ambulance crews are flat out, who communicates with the Comms centre? Nowadays, paramedics are trained in triage, and major incident management. They practice in the classroom, the outdoor scenario and real incident, and they group with other ambos, doctors and nurses to hone their skills. But in the early days of my career journey all this was done by MO1. They were requested to attend all the Gucci jobs; stabbings, shootings, road accidents, hangings, train crashes, and anything else that involved multiple casualties or serious injury. I used to think that any budding trauma junky would have given their right arm for this job, although as I was later to find out, the role was not actually clinical, but more a management one. In any case, in my early days, I had neither the experience or the qualification to even contemplate such a thing.

In 1988, Mr Keith Porter, (later to become Professor Sir Keith Porter) trauma and consultant orthopaedic surgeon, formed the CARE Team. The Central Accident Resuscitation and Extrication team, was initially a voluntary partnership between Mr Porter and West Midlands Ambulance Service whereby doctors would be available to provide their expertise in the pre hospital field to assist the ambulance crews and improve patient care. In return the doctors could tap into a wealth of trauma and medical emergencies, thereby gaining experience and furthering their own development. So everybody benefited; the crews, the doctors, and more importantly, the patients. As the years have progressed, the CARE Team has gone from strength to strength and now have official charitable status, thanks to a full time paid manager.

The partnership saw an extra Mike Oscar vehicle which was needed to transport the team, consisting of a doctor, a nurse, an observer who was usually a qualified doctor training in the pre hospital field, and finally a paramedic who both drove and became the incident commander at serious incidents. This CARE team vehicle took on the call sign of Mike Oscar 3, which for every Friday, Saturday and Sunday evening became synonymous with attending anything of a serious or potentially serious nature. From 2003 until the end of my employment with West Midlands Ambulance Service (WMAS) in 2009, I manned the CARE team on a regular basis as the incident commander and paramedic, and had the privilege to work alongside some incredible people, who shared their knowledge for the improvement of patient care. Medical consultants, military nurses fresh back from Afghanistan, SAS medics, and nurses with more experience and pre hospital know how than any one could shake a stick at. These evening shifts were sheer entertainment; the camaraderie, the black humour, filling our faces on Chinese takeaways, attending the cream of the trauma, and getting to drive some decent cars to boot was something I looked forward to when I knew I'd secured a shift on The Team. We were supplied with a Volvo XC70 estate, 2.5 litre, 5 cylinder turbo diesel with loads of room for all the kit and generally all the power needed to effortlessly perform. I felt the same levels of excitement, the same adrenaline rush, and rekindled those butterflies I'd felt all those years ago when riding third man with the crews from Henrietta street. The Team provided more tales of woe, blood, humour and destruction to feed my literary needs.

Humour is a big thing in many environments which see death and misery. Its use has been documented and well known to be a form of coping mechanism for people who regularly experience this kind of thing, and The CARE Team was no different. Done strictly away from the scene and never in front of any unlike minded individuals, it was often the raw, vulgar, piss-taking variety especially if any one member was military, and sometimes it was more of a gentlemanly type.

One cold, dark Saturday evening, the team consisted of Sharon, then my girlfriend and a very capable, experienced nurse who's never phased by anything, and somehow always seems to fathom the answers to any problem, and a very close couple of friends of ours, Dr Raul Davis, and his fiancee Dr Cate Orton. Raul was a senior registrar anaesthetist and hugely capable in the pre-hospital field. His skills were ideal within the Team, as many really sick patients needed advanced airway management and general anaesthesia. And his mannerisms fitted well; boyish sometimes immature humour when it was appropriate, and fiercely serious professionalism when the jobs demanded. With Raul, one minute we'd be laughing raucously at some childish joke, the next he'd be bollocking me for talking and disturbing his concentration when anaesthetising a fitting patient. Once he'd put a patient to sleep, then paralysed them, if he couldn't secure an airway, that patient was as good as dead. When Raul asked for quiet, he demanded quiet. Consequently, the word 'fuck' was used in all its guises on a frequent basis. Cate on the other hand was less experienced, but still an incredible doctor, and above all a very humanistic person, with a wonderful bedside manner, and a wicked sense of humour that made her fit in well.

One Saturday evening, things had been going somewhat slow for The Team. We'd had a couple of jobs, but nothing of note. Sat on the garage forecourt of the Jet petrol station alongside Hockley's cemetery, we pondered on whether this evening would produce anything 'decent'. There had been a period of silence in the car where I for one had a blank expression as I stared out to the passing traffic. What is it that makes a completely bizarre and random thought pop into our heads at times like these? I began to voice mine.

"When I was 17, me and my brother Simon had a burping

competition....", Cate piped up mid sentence.

"Why does that not surprise me, if your brother is anything like you?" I continued.

"Yeah, well it all went a bit tits up too. We were sat in my car and he came up with this gloriously funny idea of necking a can of Pepsi, then seeing who could do the loudest, longest belch. It was a bit one sided really because he went first, and after drinking it all in one go, he leaned forward, turned his head at an angle and contorted his face." At this point I imitated the way I saw him, and continued. "He stated that he felt really sick, then started an enormous belch, which very soon erupted into projectile vomiting. Pepsi came down his nose, and out of his mouth as he proceeded to throw up sticky brown liquid all over the dash of my bloody car. I never did get rid of the sickly smell". Recounting the story, for me, had been funny enough, but Cate and Raul started laughing. Sharon soon joined them with some comment agreeing with Cate that she wasn't in the least bit surprised knowing Simon. During the commotion, I spoke up with an idea.

"Why don't we have a CARE Team burping competition?" The others agreed, and I laid out the rules. "Right, first up, it has to be Pepsi...." Sharon protested.

"Yuk, I will vomit if I have to drink Pepsi. Can I drink lemonade?"

"Hmmm, well, it's not in the rule book," I replied, "and you're gonna be at a disadvantage because lemonade's not so fizzy, but yeah ok." Raul developed a childish giggle and suggested we had two categories; loudness and longevity. And so it was agreed.

We went into the garage and purchased our weapons. Three cans of Pepsi and a can of lemonade. The rules were discussed and agreed upon. It was boys against girls, but drinking a full can was a little difficult, so it was up to the individual contestant to drink as much as they thought necessary to produce the desired winning entry. Besides, if any of us had the same result as Simon, all those years ago, it wouldn't be pretty. Raul went first drinking about half the can. We all looked on waiting for the birth of something enormous, eyes and mouths agape with anticipation. Then his pathetic attempt came to fruition. Small burps consecutively but nothing of any significance. Raul seemed pleased with his attempt. The girls booed and I looked at him in disgust.

"Is that the best you can do Raul?"

"Yeah well," he started, "I'm not used to this sort of thing. I've led a very sheltered upbringing you know."

"Well you should be ashamed, and not surprised if you don't get asked to rejoin the team next year". Sharon shouted up from the back of the car.

"Well go on then, see if you can do any better." I also drank about half the can, waited the statutory few seconds then distorted my face to ease the passage of gas up. It started, and continued for a couple of seconds before stopping. I was pleased with my effort, and received some praise from the girls in the rear.

"Yeah, not bad," said Cate. " But my turn now. She duly drank most of the can, which straight away got me concerned for such a slightly framed woman. Raul, realising he'd let the side down, sat in the front and adopted a childlike pose with arms folded and a statue-like stare out of the window, refusing to take part anymore. We waited, again with eager anticipation. But nothing happened. For what seemed like an age, she remained quiet, just looking at me. She was even able to speak, a skill which impressed me no end. Then, following an eternity, she looked me in the eye, and in a very gentle, feminine tone, spoke.

"Here it comes". She let forth the most incredible burp. It just went on for ages. We reckoned a good five seconds, and one which would surely get her into the England rugby squad.

"Bloody hell Cate. That's put me in the shade hasn't it?" I said with despondence. She gave me a satisfied grin before sitting back obviously revelling in her success. She turned to Sharon.

"Your turn Sharon", as she pulled the ring on the can of lemonade and handed it over. Sharon's never been very good at drinking huge quantities of liquid, so I was banking on still potentially securing the loudest burp, as we'd agreed following Cate's gargantuan effort, that mine had been louder but much shorter. Sharon sheepishly put the can to her lips and started drinking. I'd reckoned she'd managed only about a quarter of the can before she stopped. It was in the bag for me, or so I thought until she burped forth, the loudest one I've ever heard. It shook the car! Not of any credible length, but oh my, was it loud. And so the boys had lost.

Raul was still sulking when the radio called out our call sign.

"Metro Mike Oscar 3, Mike Oscar 3 you receiving?". I picked up the microphone and acknowledged. They continued. "We have an RTA for you, M5 south bound junction one to two. Unsure what's going on at the moment, but believed serious with a potential fatal. We've had several calls on this one and an early response and update would be appreciated." I confirmed the details, as the mood in the car went from immature to professional. Laughing stopped and planning started. I knew where we were, and I knew where we needed to be. On went the blue lights and the seat belts and off we went. Raul and the girls discussed who was to carry out which role on scene. My job was always constant; communications, updates, resource planning and safety, but the rest of the team took it in turns to lead the clinical aspect of triage, assessment and treatment. This gave fantastic developmental exposure to the nurses who were traditionally pushed aside if there was a doctor on scene.

The media glorify driving under emergency conditions as being glamorous, easy and exciting. It carries an incredible degree of responsibility for the driver, their passengers and other road users, and driving style and speed should be consistent for all cases, regardless of the details of the case being driven to. The driver should drive as fast as is safe, and if that means it's dangerous to exceed ten miles an hour driving down a road with children having just come out of school, then so be it. In this case I had a 12 mile journey to get to the M5. And at the sort of speeds that traffic conditions allowed, the sirens went on when we left and were switched off on scene.

We got to junction one within a few minutes and proceeded southbound, but quickly realised that the incident was behind us on the same carriageway, prior to the junction. This meant having to get off at junction two, turn round and come all the way back, bypassing junction one, to the next point where we could turn around and come back up behind the incident. This delayed us by around five minutes but couldn't be helped.

There were other emergency vehicles already on scene but by too short a margin to have been able to give a sitrep of exact location. Incidents on motorways, particularly serious ones, are classically identified by the backing up of traffic, and this one was no different. About half a mile of stationary traffic meant the only way through was to traverse the hard shoulder. Although it was dark, this section of the motorway was illuminated with street lamps, and under the yellow glow, as we approached, I saw a stationary coach in lane one and several cars parked in all three lanes but not near each other. Initially we were puzzled, as it didn't appear that any of the vehicles had collided with each other. There were no crumpled bonnets, no steam coming from broken radiators and no cars on their roofs. Only people standing around in groups, out of the their cars, some with hands in their pockets.

The emergency services were by now arriving in droves as the respective control rooms had perceived this one as being something worthy of sending everything they had. Fire trucks, police traffic units, traffic control units, paramedic responders, ambulances and us. The sea of blue lights over powered the yellow glow of the street lamps as we arrived on scene. My initial task was to park our vehicle in such a way as to provide safety in the form of a barrier between us dealing with the patient, and any oncoming vehicles, but get us close enough to facilitate the use of all the equipment we carry, as much of it may have been needed in a hurry. Switching off the siren, and slowing the car towards a stop, I could see a large area of lane three where there were neither cars nor people; instead a large tarpaulin sheet lay on the road, the bump in the middle usually signifying a body underneath. We'd decided en route that Colly was to lead this one, and as I positioned the Volvo into the fend off position some metres back from the tarpaulin, the mood in our car seemed strangely quiet and sombre.

A coach had taken a full load of football fans to Manchester. En route they had been a little rowdy but had been without issue as the cans of beer had started flowing. However, by the time the driver picked them up after the match, the alcohol had taken its toll, along with winning the match and now they were out of hand. Abusive shouting, singing and dancing in the isle had forced the driver to continually ask for them to settle down, to which they had refused. Time after time he had politely asked down the microphone for his passengers to behave, remain seated, and keep the noise down, but with little success. His tone became firmer to the point where he lost his patience and cool, and with some annoyance, as they entered the M5, he shouted over the tannoy that he was pulling off at the next junction to call the Police, and where the rowdy mob would be thrown off. One man, decided otherwise, and allegedly turned and shouted down to the driver from the aisle where he'd been dancing and shouting.

"Don't wait until then mate, I'm fuckin' gettin' off 'ere....". His comments went unheard by the driver who by now was still in lane two, mentally preparing to leave at the next exit. The man, naked from the waist up, proceeded towards the rear of the coach, pushing past others who were standing in the isle. When he reached the back seat, he grabbed the handle of the emergency exit, and without so much of a hesitation turned it, opened the door, and jumped out into the middle lane at 70 miles per hour.

Traffic was heavy on this section of the motorway, as the evening progressed. It was cold but visibility was aided by the yellow haze of the street lighting on this section. A small hatchback had been driving northbound in an unremarkable journey. It had been following the coach for several miles as their speeds matched. The coach overtook, the hatchback overtook. The coach pulled into lane one, so did the car, and keeping a reasonable following distance, the driver noticed people standing in the isle, many of them with no shirts on, waving their arms and dancing as if drunk.

The driver, a casually dressed man of retiring age, noticed the coach slowing slightly, and checking his drivers side mirror, indicated and moved into the middle lane to overtake the long vehicle. When he was a matter of ten meters behind and rapidly approaching, the rear emergency door opened, and a semi clothed male jumped out with some deliberation. It all happened so quickly, and faster than physical human reaction could occur. The driver remembered seeing it, almost in slow motion, as it's often described, but was paralysed to do anything about it. Something large hit his bonnet, and it quickly became apparent it was a person; arms and legs flailing, a momentary view of a face, hair, something red smearing the windscreen as it stoved it in and crazed the glass so the driver lost his view, as it disappeared over the roof of the car. The driver instinctively slammed the brakes on without thought of following vehicles, and from way back the southbound lane became a sea of red lights as everybody reacted and braked.

The Alton family had also been proceeding in the same direction, and had been following the small hatchback moments before. They had had an equally uneventful journey in their people carrier, and too had noticed what appeared to be rowdy behaviour inside the coach verbally remarking so. Mr Alton, driving, did not see the emergency exit of the coach open. Instead, his first involvement was seeing something come from the roof of the car in front, land in the road between them, prior to him driving over whatever it was with a double 'bump' in rapid succession. Not seeing exactly what it was, he initially thought it a bicycle having come off a car in front, however, his suspicions changed as he drove over it, describing it as something softer than a bicycle. And after he'd driven over the football fan, so the vehicle behind also did, until eventually, all the vehicles had come to a stop fairly quickly. The whole event had taken a matter of seconds, and now, straddling lanes two and three, lay the football fan. No dancing, no singing and no shouting. Instead he lay motionless.

In these circumstances, my initial role was one of safety. Just because all vehicles appeared to be stationary, didn't mean than a member of my team wasn't at risk of being hit by a stray member of the public 'rubber necking', or indeed another emergency vehicle whose driver wasn't paying full attention. I had to keep my eye on all three of them, all of the time, and the distinctive high visibility one piece suits worn by members of the CARE Team did make life a little easier for me. Nobody alights the vehicle until the incident commander gives the go ahead, and once I was happy, I gave the order, telling the guys to be careful and keep a watchful eye out.

As my role wasn't primarily a clinical one, Sharon, Cate and

Raul made their way to the tarpaulin sheet, while I liaised with other emergency staff and members of the public, to ascertain just what we were dealing with here, and how many casualties we had. A police officer gave me a very brief run down of events and aside of the car occupants who had hit the football fan being badly shaken and upset, our only serious casualty lay in the road before us. I made my way to the team who were by now crouching on the floor alongside the covered bump, starting to peer underneath. A large crowd had now developed, as people uninvolved in the incident, but caught up in the traffic jam had left their cars and vans and walked forward, standing in a line some 20 meters away, held back by the police, but in clear view of what lay before us. In cases such as these, sheeting is most usually placed over the casualty for one reason, and one reason only; and we have to be mindful not to uncover things in view of the onlookers in such circumstances. Therefore, I utilised the services of a couple of firemen to stand on the side of the tarpaulin nearest the onlookers, so that when lifted, the sheeting would shield the sight. All members of the public forward of our position were also sent back towards the crowd to for their own visual protection.

As the sheet was lifted, it was messy. A deceased male lay before us with massive cranial destruction. The left side of his face was pressed into the Tarmac, his jaw dislocated and virtually ripped out of the skull revealing teeth and bone, and a distortion to his cheeks. His right eye had partly avulsed and moving my vision upwards, the occipital region of the back of his skull was almost completely missing, where upon brain tissue had exploded under pressure and was spread in a line across the tarmac for some meters. All four limbs were severely and compoundly fractured, sending them in unnatural directions, and the whole upper torso was blanketed in gravel rash and had a dirty look about it, as if it had been dragged around a field for days. It was obvious that this poor man hadn't suffered. He'd died an instant death.

Raul had already approached the upset and shocked car occupants to see if they needed anything, leaving the girls and myself with the body. There was somehow an eerie level of, not silence, but quiet that seemed to cocoon the three of us behind our tarpaulin sheet, allowing us to get on with the grisly task in hand. To us, this was fascinating; a live lesson in anatomy, and wild guesses as to what killed him first. With the two girls crouching beside the body, and me onlooking, Sharon turned to Colly.

"As you're more senior than me, you'll have to confirm death on the body Cate." Cate looked up at Sharon with somewhat of a mild concern on her face.

"But I've never done one pre hospitally before....." She said, hesitating momentarily, then speaking again for clarification of the process of death confirmation, but phrased it somewhat inaccurately. "So how do I know he's dead...", as she looked up at Sharon for advice. I too looked at Sharon now with a grin developing on my face, because I knew what was coming. Sharon returned the look to Cate with a serious expression. The look in her eye gave away a glint of black humour. In a hushed voice she spoke.

"Well, when a patient's brains are sitting between my knees, but not inside his head, and his skull is between your hands and not attached to his body I think it's safe to say he's dead." My grin grew into one of those moments when stifling a laugh becomes difficult, and I sensed the other two were experiencing the same. Cate returned fire with a hushed voice.

"Yeah I know that you cheeky cow, I mean what's the process?" Sharon and I regained our composure for the sake of professionalism, and between us we explained.

The normal process of confirming death includes checking for a carotid pulse, the presence of breathing and heart sounds, a central response and finally the eyes for pupil reaction. However, in this case, massive cranial destruction bypasses some of these to simplify the process. Death confirmed, and the sheeting was replaced. In cases like these, the scene is one of a criminal nature until otherwise proven, and so the ambulance service withdraw leaving the police and the coroners officers to clear up the mess and reopen the road network.

Our task here was done. This job, although gruesome, had been pretty simple and straight forward. One predominant casualty, very obviously deceased, and all other folk at scene needing pre hospital care being dealt with by the other attending paramedics. There is sometimes a desire to stay on scene to soak up more of the atmosphere, but I'd decided our time was best spent with the living elsewhere, so gathering the team back to the car, I booked us available.

CHAPTER 30. BRUCE LEE IN THE MAKING.

The great thing about working with the Central Accident Resuscitation and Extrication Team, known simply as the 'CARE' Team, was the sheer variety of people who manned it, all bringing their own mix of experience, qualifications, style and character. It wasn't all clinical. One regular attender to the team was Al Sartori. I'd always assumed his first name was actually Alec or Alan and was surprised to learn some years later that his name was Alouicious Sartori. His origins lay in the wealthy Sartori family of Messina, Sicily, who made their wealth in the citrus and olive groves, but he was a Londoner through and through, born and raised in Hackney. Al was a well travelled man, and although not in academic terms, he had more real term experience of the front line and reality than anyone I've met before or since. His full time job, was that of police officer. Not just any old police officer. He was part of the close protection guys, of which we'll delve no further, suffice to say that he was an expert in weighing people up, from a criminal perspective. If he came across someone who was about to be up to no good, Al knew it before the crime was committed. He just had a nose for it. In his spare time, he trained and qualified as a paramedic. And a nurse. Oh, and a squaddie in the Territorial army. His rather extravagant heritage saw him with unusual middle names of Nelson Ulysses, but he never used them and was just known as Al. Or more precisely to me, Big Al.

Al was a big bloke. Six foot something, with hands like shovels and the strength of Goliath. It wasn't his size that I found interesting. It was the way he communicated, the way he could fathom situations, and just his sheer level of common sense. In all the time I've known him, only on a very few occasions has his size and strength been needed. For his intuition and perception was used as an incredible weapon. His military humour just kept coming and coming......

I first met Al in my earlier days on The CARE Team. Arriving to start my shift, we were despatched to an entrapment RTC in Dudley before I'd even had a chance to check the car. Al sat in the back quietly, next to a fresh faced doctor chap, whilst Ashley Goodruth, a guy who fulfilled the nurse position who I knew quite well, sat next to me in the front. Al had been mates with Ash for some time, and had been introduced to work on The Team by him. As the job had come in quickly I'd not really even had chance to look at Al before setting off, merely knowing that he was there. Birmingham to Dudley took us the best part of 20 minutes under emergency driving conditions, and by the time we'd arrived the fire service were well under way to cutting the car into numerous pieces to extract the patient, who from my perspective did not seem life threatening, making his entrapment what is termed 'relative'.

The local ambulance crew had been in attendance for some time before us and seemed to have the case sorted, meaning our role was to take a back stance and watch from the side lines, so to speak. Ash, being hugely experienced and confident, headed The Team for the evening as the doctor was new in to the pre hospital field, and had the feel about him of the 'new boy'. He'd been encouraged forward into the thick of the road accident to gain a bit of experience of the anatomy of vehicle make up, leaving Ash, Al and myself standing next to each other, with me in the middle.

I'd still not been introduced to Al before Ash's arm came round the back of me to touch him on the shoulder.

"You're it!" Ash stated with some seriousness. I became aware of Al glaring at Ash past me, with a look on his face like he'd been dealt a bad hand. He adjusted his glare very slightly so that now he was looking directly at me. My gaze was still in the direction of the cut up car as I tried to pretend I hadn't noticed what was going on between the two of them. Then without warning, Al stuck his finger in my ear, and screwed it back and forth a few times as if trying to deposit something from his finger into the orifice.

"I'm Al", he stated. "And you're it." I turned to him.

"I'm what?" I replied with an air of bewilderment. His face remained forward and serious, as he spoke out of the corner of his mouth nearest to me.

"You've never played 'Poo tig' have you?" It was obvious to him I hadn't, so before I could answer, he explained. "Imagine I've just wiped my finger right across my arse hole having followed through. My finger now contains just a little bit of poo, and that's what I've wiped in your ear." Strangely enough, he'd now got my attention. He continued. "So now it's your turn to carry it on. But you can't wipe it back on to the person who gave it you. It has to be someone else."

Hearing this, Ash walked away, and towards the doctor, as if he was actually going to advise him, or perform something clinical on the patient. It was however, obvious to me he didn't want to be poo tigged. This type of immature humour was common place on the front line with many. The secret is to know when it's appropriate, and when it's not, and to ensure that no one, but no one around you has any idea of what's going on.

Al was right; I'd never taken part in such frivolities, but

keeping my cool, remaining stationary for just long enough to throw suspicion, I sidled over to Ash, who, as he leaned forward to check on the doctor, had a couple of words whispered in his ear and a finger smeared across his upper lip from behind. I stepped back and turned to look at Al, who of course by now was developing a smirk, and an evasive counter plan knowing that Ash would shortly be heading in his direction. And so began the friendship of an incredible bloke.

Another regular game played within The CARE team environment, didn't have a name but involved the insertion of a word within a sentence. This word had to be from a chosen group such as a musical instrument or an animal, decided upon at the start of the shift, and for each word stated, score would be retained, one point for each word. The sentence had to be within communication to the patient, a relative, another doctor at the hospital etc. So for example, if the chosen group was animals and we attended a patient with mobility issues, such as a twisted ankle and who couldn't walk well, someone might be heard to say, "So, you're not as fast as a gazelle today are you?" Or perhaps the patient with a sore throat and laryngitis might asked how long their voice has been horse." I'm sure you get the picture……

I'd only completed a few shifts with the Team, but already I was hooked into an arena which threw a hearty mix of adrenaline, excitement, fear, blood and a large dollop of clinical development in my direction, because we generally attended only those cases that required the specialism of a doctor, expert in the pre-hospital field. Birmingham's one million population created shootings, hangings, rapes, mutilation, crashes, traumatic amputations and stabbings. Lots of stabbings. And we got to deal with many of them.

April 2004, saw me get a phone call to confirm my shifts with The Team for the next few months. They were always performed on overtime, but for me, I couldn't get enough of it. At the time I was working Monday to Friday office hours, so the Team shifts of Friday, Saturday and Sunday evenings, fell into my off time. Perfect for overtime. To think I was doing something with which I had an incredible passion and gave me immense satisfaction, and they were paying me for the privilege.

The summer evenings on The Team always brought cases of incredible diversity. Some of the most memorable road accidents, train decapitations, shootings and general human mutilation seemed to have been when folk ventured out into the warm, long, light evenings, where many of them wouldn't be seeing the following morning. Alcohol, of course, often played a pivotal role in their demise, as did socio-economic status; the lower the status of an area, and the more densely populated, so the more chance we would find ourselves up to our eyeballs in guts and bullets. I worked with some incredible people; nurses, doctors and military medics who demonstrated undeniable skill and ability, many of whom I still keep in touch with today, many years on.

Josephine Hanna was an upcoming doctor who'd recently earned her wings to work on the Team as the doc. This is no mean feat. Aside of their medical qualifications and experience, they had to be mentored on the road by one of the senior Team doctors who were often consultants in anaesthetics or emergency medicine. Their tough assessments ensured that any doctor they put their name to, was ready to operate independently.

We all liked Jo. She had a bubbly, 'normal' personality that immediately put everyone at ease. She spoke to everyone at their own level and always really cared for the person she was talking to. I always put this down to her background, coming from an ordinary working class family, so she'd not seen the wealth or the lavish lifestyle. Some doctors on the Team had a persona of total intellect, and found the team not easy to acclimatise to, and the team's black humour and constant, appropriate laughter made these types less able to fit in. But Jo fitted in well. A larger than average girl, she'd started using the gym in a bid to reduce weight and get back into a fit she'd had as a teenager. It turned out that she was once very slim and fit, and had taken up karate, of which she'd achieved a black belt. No mean feat and something which impressed us on the team the day she told us.

It was nearing 9 o'clock on a cold autumn evening, and I'd been looking forward to this shift for a while because Al Sartori was working it. Jo was the doctor, on one of her first independent evenings, and the fourth space had been vacant as a medical student had pulled out at the last minute. Big Johns, the takeaway chain, was a regular haunt of The Team for food, and this evening was no exception. Parked on the side of the road, the inside of the car stank of hot chicken wings and tikka masala, and for one, I was grateful of the extra helpings of hand wipes we'd been given, seeing as how I seemed to be wearing more of the food than I'd eaten. Whilst eating, we'd been having a discussion about how fit health workers needed to be. Jo was a modest woman, and contributed to the discussion.

"Well even though I have a black belt in Karate, it was some time ago and I'm no where near as fit as I was then." Al wasn't a slim bloke and had the build of a rugby player.

"Well darlings, I love me food, but in a foot chase, he better have his running shoes on, I can tell ya." I laughed.

"Have to say Al, I wouldn't like to be on the receiving end of you in a foot chase."

"Then Bradders, don't nick anything or be a bad boy, and I won't chase ya". The conversation cut short with the phone ringing.

The Team phone generally rings when one of two things happen. There's a major incident, or they have a hum drum job they can't cover with an ambulance. Anything in between comes over the radio.

"Mike Oscar 3," I answered. "Hi Dave, it's Kerry. Could you do us a favour and have a look at a case for us? It's only a welfare check and you're pretty near to it." We were not on the road for this sort of thing, as being tied up with something minor meant we were potentially not available if something more appropriate came in. Sometimes, Control would try and use us for this type of thing frequently until we got the powers that be in to stop it some months before. But the current Comms girls were great and looked after us, so one good turn deserves another.

"Yeah no worries, Kerry. Looks like tonight is a slow starter anyway.

"Thanks guys" she said, and continued. "We've had a call from a worried lady in Bristol who can't get her brother to answer the phone. He's apparently wheelchair bound and has 24 hour carers who also aren't answering the phone. Could you check it out for us?" She gave us the address, which was indeed very local, and the remainder of the chips were rolled into their paper and put in the spare seat in the back of the car next to Al, who, as I put my seat belt on, was finishing licking his fingers.

We pulled into the street; a crescent with a large round grassed area in the middle. This part of town was not the best. Mainly council housing with an adornment of settees and old engines sat on the front gardens. In the warm summer evenings the sound of barking dogs filled the gaps between children's screams and the boom boom of loud music from upstairs open windows. But this was the chilly autumn, and at this time in the evening the place seemed pretty quiet. Driving slowly past the numbers, the soft squeak of the brakes denoted we had found ours and the car came to a halt. We surveyed the house. This one was a little more upmarket with a block paved front and a Rover car parked up towards the front door. Dried out shabby hanging baskets hung either side of the door, which a few months before had blushed with colour. The front door was a standard council type; wooden with a semi circle of glass towards the top, and red in colour. Al was the first to question if this was the correct house as there were no lights on. His question was deemed a rhetorical one.

"You guys stay here and finish the chips. It'll be the wrong address I'll bet." I said as I climbed out and gently shut the drivers door. As I walked towards the front door, the expected dog bark hit me from the other side of next door's fence, resembling something pretty big, and took me by surprise. The whirring sound of an electric car window signalled a comment from Al.

"I think he likes you……go give him a pat." I turned to give Al the raised eyebrow.

"Bloody glad there's something between me and it." I said continuing on to the front door and ringing the bell, which was fairly loud. Ambos like loud bells. It saves having to knock. I waited, then turned my ear towards the door for any sound of someone approaching the other side. Nothing. I rang again, this time holding my finger on the button so as to wake the dead. Still nothing. So I rang Kerry back to confirm the address.

"No it's definitely the correct one Dave. Hang on I'll call the sister back, hold the line".

Al and Jo, now having finished the feed got out of the car to join me to see what the score was. Still holding the phone, I told them Kerry was checking with the sister, when Kerry came back.

"Hello Dave? Nope it's definitely the right address and the

brother is in there in a wheel chair. The sister sounded really concerned." Now the excitement of breaking into a house came into play.

"Right, we'll gain access now, and if you can ask the police to attend please, that'd be good". Al popped around the back and I knocked the next house adjoining, both without success, so out came the trusty crowbar from the back of the car. Being the copper, and the biggest of the three of us, the duty of gaining access naturally fell to him. Until Jo piped up with a childish glint in her eye like she was asking mum for a lick of the cake spoon.

"Can I kick the door in Al? Please? I've always wanted to do it."

There is something particularly appealing about breaking into houses as a paramedic. Perhaps it's the wanton damage one can inflict, or the 'get out of jail free' card giving immunity from prosecution on charitable and humanitarian grounds. Or perhaps, bizarrely, it's being able to play burglars for the evening. In cases such as these the objective was to cause minimal damage, and started with a common sense approach of trying the door handle first to see if it was unlocked! A quick look around the back for an open door or window, then a knock on the neighbours door, as they often had keys to fetch shopping and supplies for house bound unfortunates. Failing that, we'd break the smallest window, to then reach in and lift a catch, or shoulder a flimsy back door that looked like it wouldn't object.

Many years before whilst riding third man with the Sutton crew of Turbo and Sticky, we'd been called to a similar case of a concerned neighbour worried about the old chap across the road, and following a few unanswered knocks on the front door, Sticky peered through the letter box where upon he saw a pair of horizontal legs jutting out from a doorway, accompanied with a moaning sound he couldn't make out.

"Bloody hell, there's a bloke collapsed in the hallway. I'll kick the front door in," and with that the large framed Sticky took a good run up and with his size 11 Doc Martins not only opened the front door but kicked it clean off its hinges so that it flew half way up the hallway nearly colliding with the legs, closely followed by bricks, splintered wood and dust. Lots of dust. As we all piled in and stood over the legs, there was a chap, upper body in the lounge, comfortably propped up on some pillows eating a sandwich. He looked at us with great surprise.

"Did you come round the back? Maud left it open for you......" I rest my case.....

Al turned to Jo, then to me.

"The crowbar is much easier." But Jo pleaded with us both.

"Oh please please, go on let me. I'm a black belt in Karate. Please?" I had no problem with it.

"Yep go ahead then. Do yer best" I said.

The front door had a standard type lock on the right side at eye height which was locked, and a handle at waist level which wasn't as I'd already tried it. Al crouched down and using the crowbar hooked it over the handle to pull it down. One less thing to create resistance. Jo stood for a second and eyed the door up. She couldn't take much of a run up, because of the car parked about 2 metres from the door. Al reminded her to kick high, where the lock was. She scowled at him

"I know. D'ya think I'm stupid?" Al spoke under his breath.

"......just saying like". She stood in front of the door, and took a pace back until her legs were up against the car bumper, turned slightly to the left then leapt forward with all she'd got, shouting forth something resembling 'hi....ya' as her right leg made contact with the door. It became obvious to all that it had been some time since she'd performed a high kick, and Jo wasn't quite as supple as when she'd regularly been practicing the martial arts. Her leg struck far too low, at the springiest part of the door, firing her back from whence she came and landing her backside straight in the middle of the bonnet, clearly having taken her by surprise judging by the wail that she let forth. My immediate reaction was to look at Jo as she slid off the bonnet, which now revealed a large dent in its middle, then my snigger started and as I looked at Al, his eyes rolled upwards as he too started to giggle, and did no more than stand up, mutter "oops slipped" as the crowbar went through the small half round window in the door. He reached in through the broken glass and undid the catch from the inside, so before Jo had even had time to stand back up again, the door was open. His timing was perfect, and added all the more to the humour.

Being dark inside the house, I went in first with torchlight, found a light switch and called out.

"Hello? Hello? Anyone home?" And with no reply I asked Al and Jo to have a look downstairs. "If there's a wheelchair here, that's where it's gonna be". I went upstairs although no bulb in the landing light meant the torch came back out.

The door at the top of the stairs was open and on the far wall was a bed with someone in it. A male, aged about 40 I'd guessed, unkempt and in need of a shave. The room was a heavy mix of alcohol, dirt and unwashed clothing, which combined to contort my face in disgust at the smell. The floor was littered with empty beer cans and rubbish. Of more concern were empty tablet foils, which on closer inspection revealed them as once having housed Diazepam, a sedative and muscle relaxant. Many years of experience has taught me that when someone with alcohol on board is woken, approach with caution and have an escape route. I shouted down the stairs for my backup.

"Al, up here". I shook the sleeping man's arm at length and spoke. No response made me shake and shout harder, still with no response, but his loud snoring confirmed to me that at least he was breathing. With Al now coming up the stairs, I gripped the mans ear lobe between my thumb and forefinger and squeezed it to initiate a pain stimulus to see if that roused him. "HELLO MATE" I shouted. He stirred, and in the blink of an eye shot out of bed and took a wild, drunken punch at me.

"Who the fuck are you?" He said in a slurred Glaswegian tone. Stepping back and avoiding the hit, I put my palms up to him in a calming gesture.

"Whooooaaaa mate, it's the ambulance service, just checking if you're ok." But this guy wasn't having any of it. I knew it, and Al, now behind me, sensed it too. The man lurched at us, but being totally unable to coordinate his movements fell flat on his face between us as we stepped aside. Al has got a fantastic way of being able to convince these type of people that he's helping them, when in fact he's actually restraining them, so to the onlooker, it all looks good. Which is what Jo thought as she came up the stairs to see the man now facing the wall, lying on the bed shouting obscenities, while his arms were pinned behind his back leaving him totally unable to do anything but shout.

Jo's face was a picture as she stood there in the door way mouth a gape.

"Did you find our man in the wheelchair Jo?" She snapped out of her stare

"Er yeah, he's downstairs in the back. He's fine." The man on the bed changed his tack, turned his head towards the door, and started on Jo.

"And who the fuck are you......? Let me fuckin' ge' a' ya fuckin' wankerrrrs. I'll fuckin' kill the lotta ya.......wankers". But there was no way he was getting out of his human handcuffs.

I made a call to confirm where the police were and stepped up the urgency. Within minutes an approaching siren hailed the arrival of the cavalry, and after handing over chummy and explaining the issue of the man downstairs, we egressed to the car for what we all knew was going to be a humorous debrief. A few seconds of silence preceded Al piping up.

"So errrrr, Jo, what style of martial......" She shut him off quickly with a growing smile.

"Don't bloody start. Oh and can we keep this to ourselves?" It's that point when, at the back of the church on a Sunday morning you've had to stifle a laugh for so long, and now the sermon is over and you're in the graveyard laughing your socks off. The laughter came in floods of tears, as they streamed down my face trying to recount the story, but somehow just couldn't get the words out.

Within a few minutes, calm was beginning to return to the inside of the car, sat out on the road under the street lights. We could hear raised voices coming from the open front door of the house, and before too long they got louder as our drunken 'carer' came out with his hands behind his back flanked by a couple of bobbies. As he walked past the car he halted making the officers turn. He looked at the bonnet, then up at his escorts.

"Look at my fuckin' car! Some fuckers' vandalised it. You bastards should be out lookin' for whoever did this. Fuckin' place is getting worse I'm fuckin' tellin ya...." They firmed their hold and forced him towards the waiting police van. As ever, Al's tone broke our concentration.

"Ee's right ya know. This place is getting worse. Fancy someone dentin' 'is bonnet like that. Must be a mob a Bruce Lees goin' round...."

CHAPTER 31 - THE PLAN THAT DIDN'T GO TO PLAN

Statistically, around the mid 1990's the chance of surviving an out-of-hospital cardiac arrest was around 4%. So, 96% of all who collapsed with a stopped heart were destined for death. This was largely due to a few factors; first off, the time taken for someone to get to the individual, recognise the severity of the their condition and call for help. Then, the time it took to get trained personnel into the scene, in the big cities with many ambulances, even 10 minutes to get to the affected was too long to save precious brain tissue from decaying to the point of no return. Then perhaps finally the difference in training of the attending medical professionals - and by this I don't put down the efficient first responder able to carry out good CPR. They were, and still are, the true life savers. Modern intervention, aside of defibrillation and certain other specialities are now known to potentially hamper survival rates of out-hospital-cardiac arrests by delaying transport to the definitive place of management, being the hospital.

We've all heard of the surviver of a cardiac arrest, because they happened to be in the right place at the right time. The man who collapsed unconscious right outside of the casualty dept, whilst visiting a sick relative (still technically an out-of-hospital incident), or the individual who collapsed on an aircraft at 35000 feet, which by coincidence was also passengered by a fleet of doctors, nurses and paramedics returning from a cardiac disease conference. And the man who collapsed into arrest literally underneath a defibrillator in a shopping centre, whilst standing next to a security guard trained in its use. These three examples are actual true events, and although technically dead, were brought back and made a full recovery - that is they survived to discharge from hospital with the ability to lead a relatively normal life. Many initial survivors of cardiac arrest, go on to become cardiac invalids, with only a small percentage of their heart muscle remaining, causing them to be unable to exert themselves to virtually any extent without developing severe breathlessness and chest pain, and often die a short time later from complications such as heart failure.

Modern ways have attacked this problem in a few ways. More responding health professionals, better geographically placed to access emergencies, defibrillators spread all over the community with people trained to use them, and a heightened awareness of the public through education of the issue. The right resource, to the right patient, at the right time, so to speak.

One aspect of working on the front line for many years, was that I developed an intimate geographical and topographical knowledge of the areas in which I worked. Once inhabited by the rich and affluent, one inner city area had inner city problems. Crime and unemployment were fairly high and the place wasn't regarded as being the most desirable of areas. With a bustling ethnic mix and diverse culture, it was always a hive of activity.

Delroy was a young man of 26. He'd had his fair share of life troubles; kicked out of school after school, he was arrested several times as a teenager for cannabis issues, petty theft and assault. And as time went on he spent time in prison, and used this opportunity in the gym. Consequently, he was a well built guy with muscle who liked to show it off wearing singlets topped off with plenty of bling in the form of gold chains 'Mr T' style. He struggled with intellect and found himself getting frustrated with others who didn't understand his needs, leading to more violence and more police custody. He'd had a string of girlfriends over the years who came and went and probably a few children too, of which he had neither contact or concern. His alcoholic father beat him mercilessly as a child while his mother, powerless to intervene, stood by, and having been brought up in a life of violence and hardship, the theme continued. Many, if not all the girlfriends were assaulted on a regular basis through out their relationship with him. Although there was no denying he was a good looking lad, who initially had a way with the ladies, he was a typical bully, preying on those weaker, and once they got wind of his ways, the girls would leave him. Unable to hold down, or even want a job, he drew the dole, making more money small time dealing drugs to the locals. He had been referred for counselling on several occasions but had always either dropped out, or been discharged through his behaviour. The authorities reckoned they could lead a horse to water.... and all that.

Samantha was a stunningly attractive girl of 5"8' with a beautiful complexion. Slim and in her mid 20's, she was intelligent and had done well at school, earning a good job with a big firm of solicitors in the city, where she'd been for some years. She always dressed well and came across as articulate and smart, demonstrating she had plans to further her career into something better still. You could say, she was entirely the opposite of Delroy.

Sam worked hard during the week, and as a way of relaxing, like so many people, she'd go clubbing at the weekends and let her hair down, and was always on the look out for the right guy to show her a good time. Which is how she came to meet Delroy. Dressed to impress, he had a silver tongue when it came to the ladies. Not too heavy, he had the right mix of chat and initial persona that got Sam interested. They danced, smooched and went for food on that first meeting, leaving at the end having exchanged phone numbers.

At the start, things went well. He was polite, almost a gentleman, but as he became more familiar with Sam, Delroy's old ways crept in as he tried to take possession of her, demanding to know who she'd been speaking to that day, or what text messages she'd received, occasioning going through her phone and handbag. Sam found him demanding money from her, and trying to control her daily movements. She had one factor that Delroy didn't, and neither, it would seem, did his previous relationships. Intelligence and ability to match, and counteract, his demands. She knew their relationship was destined to go nowhere, but she hung onto it. In between his attempts to control and bully, he was affectionate and sweet, with a generous side, like he'd shown for the first few months after they had met. He'd bring her flowers and chocolates after they'd quarrelled. But these weren't displays of affection; these were peace offerings, because Delroy knew for the first time in his life, he'd lost an argument. And as time went on, he found himself losing more and more. He couldn't bully Sam. He couldn't frighten her. And he couldn't have his own way. She would outwit him every time. And in the realisation that their relationship was never going to go anywhere, she finally came clean with him and told him; its over.

Delroy didn't take to rejection too well. In his mind, Sam was probably joking, or needing a bit of space. Bigger bunches of flowers and bigger boxes of chocolates would soon bring her back. Sam, however, had other ideas. Her relationship with Delroy was never that serious and was destined in her mind to never really go anywhere. He'd shown her a good time while it lasted and that was it. Delroy didn't think in this way and not knowing anything different he continued with the same actions that had retrieved many girls in the past when his demeanour and actions had sent them west. Initially he would call her often, asking for forgiveness and promising to change, but Sam had moved on. She had resumed her life and was going out with her friends continuing the hunt for good times. His calls became intrusive and he wouldn't take no for an answer so Sam stopped answering them. His tactic changed to turning up at her place of work, causing further issue, resulting in her seeking advice from the police who spoke to Delroy and warned him about his behaviour. So he figured he'd turn up the wick and resort to emotional blackmail.

Some years before, Delroy had taken tenancy of a ground floor council flat which at the time was seen as being in a low socio economic area. Crime and unemployment were high and there was a desperate need to have investment within to bring the area up. The tower block was directly opposite a police station but this didn't deter property break-ins from occurring and in an attempt to tackle this issue, the council took steps at considerable cost to improve the security of it's social housing tower blocks by installing more secure main entrance doors and intercom systems. Individual apartment doors were reinforced with steel frames, and ground and second floor windows were fitted with thick perspex and more secure frames. These improvements were welcomed by the tenants and their committees, and sure enough burglary statistics reduced. However, within days the intercom system and main entrance door had been vandalised and no longer worked, allowing all and sundry to at least enter the foyer.

One dry, sunny Saturday afternoon, having not heard from him for a few weeks, Sam's brother received a text from Delroy, who had been prohibited from making direct contact with Sam. Her brother rang her. Delroy was threatening to hang himself unless she would go round to his place and talk with him. Sam was wary and didn't know how to view the threat, as this was not something he'd done before. Guilt getting the better of her on the basis of 'what if', saw her texting Delroy telling him she would come straight round but that he better not be playing with her or she would be reporting him to the police again. She told him she'd be 30 minutes, the time it would take to drive from her place to his.

Delroy had hatched what in his mind was the perfect plan; he removed the glass panel above his kitchen door and threw a rope over the exposed frame, with a high noose. He would stand on a stereo speaker, place the rope around his neck and wait for Sam to arrive. He figured she would knock on the front door which he wouldn't answer. She would panic based on his threat of hanging himself, come around to the window where she would look in. At that point he would kick the speaker away, hang himself in front of her at which point she would rush back round, let herself in the front door, cut him down and cradle him in her arms, realising his seriousness of feelings, and they'd all live happily ever after.

Sure enough, Sam arrived, entered the foyer and knocked loudly on Delroy's front door, calling out his name, to which he didn't reply. As he'd anticipated she exited the building, ran around and peered through the window. Seeing him with his neck in the noose, Sam quickly realised he was serious and became hysterical, shouting to him not to hang himself, at which point he furthered his plan and kicked away the speaker, leaving his feet swinging and off the floor. However, Delroy's plan rapidly failed from this point, because Sam no longer had his front door key, having left it in his flat last time she was there when she told him it was over between them. Realising she now had no way in, Sam had the presence of mind to run across the road to the police station, where upon she summoned help and several officers returned within minutes. And looking through the window there he was hanging; struggling and wretching, face starting to swell and change colour. What must have been going through his mind at that point, seeing the onlooking faces and perhaps realising that his rescue might not take place at all? One of the police officers drew his baton in an attempt to smash the glass, but it bounced off the reinforcement. Again he tried. Again and again and again, frantically trying to smash the impossible, while seeing the life slip away from Delroy. His colleagues rushed to the front door in a vein attempt to kick it in. But again hampered by the steel frame. A call was made for the fire and ambulance services to attend, and within more minutes the front door was being jacked open with hydraulic force. In they rushed and supporting the weight of the now limp Delroy, they cut him down, and seeing an absence of breathing or pulse, resuscitation was commenced.

My shift on The CARE team had started that day with a road traffic accident. The report had come through of major injuries and total carnage. But as so often happens, upon arrival everybody was out of the cars involved and walking around the scene holding sore necks with minor cuts and bruising evidential, but clearly not in need of our specialised services. Hunger then predominated and a trip to 'Big Johns' was in order for perhaps a bowl of chicken tikka masala or their speciality pizza. There is an unwritten law of physics with ambos that no matter how long it has been since the last job, the next one won't come in until you're just sitting down to eat, you've ordered and paid but haven't yet received your food, you've just got in the shower, or just sat on the loo, having an enormous urge for a bowel movement that hasn't yet birthed. It happens, and it happens all, and I mean *all*, the time. In my early days at Henrietta Street Ambulance Station we used to regularly check for the camera inside the teapot because it happened then and 35 years later it still bloody does!

Big Johns had taken my money. I'd decided on the pizza, which of course is made fresh. Which takes time. A lifetime.

Loaded with chicken pieces, pineapple, cheese and all manner of delights my mouth watered as it disappeared into the depths of the oven on the moving conveyor. The further in it got, the higher my level of anxiety, knowing that the phone would ring. Sure enough, there it was! Ringing loudly, the other 3 team members turned around to face me, glaring. Despite the fact that usually we only attended the more serious cases, when I called out what the job was, it was always met with moans and groans if food had been ordered, although carried out under the breath and whilst making for the car, UNLESS it was a cardiac arrest, which prompted a seriousness of rapidity and response. I half mouthed at the others in the presence of a take away full of hungry punters "cardiac arrest" as I was already half way outside. The others followed and into the car we got, engine started, seat belts on and flat tracking to the scene a matter of 5 minutes away.

On route to these cases discussion occurs between the members as to whose role is what, often taking things in turns for awesome clinical development. On this occasion the doctor was Kieran, a portly, quietly spoken Irishman with a speciality in emergency medicine and paediatrics and a sense of humour befitting the team.The nurse was Sharon and the third seat was occupied by an army guy who I knew only as 'Inky'. The military used to come out with us on a regular basis to gain civilian trauma knowledge but with them they brought masses of experience and equipment usually only reserved for the battle setting. At the start of the shift, during equipment check, Inky had been showing me a new piece of gear the military had been using for some time but the ambulance services were yet to embrace; the Bone Injection Gun or simply the BIG. A device that fires a needle into bone to provide a point of entry for drugs and fluids where intra venous access is not possible due to venous shutdown. I remember telling Inky that during this shift, he'd got more chance of meeting The Pope than using the BIG………!

Sharon, the nurse, would lead the resuscitation if it was deemed viable. This role was almost 'hands off' and visually managing the attempt, directing others to do certain tasks, and normally doing so from a standing position at the foot of the patient. This role is so important in the instance where there is the luxury of many players at a resuscitation, and happens all the time in hospital but rarely in the prehospital setting due to lack of staff numbers. Kieran was allocated to the airway and Inky the chest compressions. My role, as ever was scene resource management, communications and extrication.

Upon arrival we were met by a police officer who quickly appraised us of the situation. These are the times where idle chat is off the cards and succinct quickly retrieved info is in; where is the patient? How long was he hanging? As he was leading us into the flat and to Delroy he estimated he'd been hanging for about 10 minutes before being cut down. Now in the lounge room, one fire fighter was performing chest compressions and another was ventilating Delroy with a bag valve mask device. I could see he was unresponsive and pale faced with evidence of cyanosis around his lips. The team got to work in that smooth, orchestrated way that I'd seen so often with prehospital care. The cardiac monitor/defibrillator was switched on and the patches applied to Delroy's chest, showing him to be in ventricular fibrillation, a life threatening cardiac rhythm needing to be defibrillated. It is the only action that could have a positive result, so it was charged and fired. With no change, it was charged and fired again and this time resolving the fibrillation and converting it to a flat line of asystole. CPR was recommenced and the suction tubing made the familiar noise that only a vomit occluded airway produces, and ventilation continued. Sharon started writing on her leg patch the times of events so key to scene management and post operative administration. The airway became Kieran's domain and was soon secured with an intubation tube, as a fire fighter took over chest compressions and Inky went for venous access. Under these clinical conditions, sometimes the patient's veins stand out like drainpipes and sometimes there's nothing to be either visualised or felt, and with experience you kind of know if you're going to have a challenge or a walk in the park.

Inky applied a venous tourniquet to the upper arm and sensed he would have trouble getting a cannula in following a rapid palpation of the dorsum and anticubital fossa. He reached for his bag and out came the BIG. This device looks like its come out of the torture chamber of the 14th century, consisting of a large syringe type mechanism with several protruding spikes arranged in a circumference. The device is place at 90° to the sternum and pushed down…hard. When all the circumferential pins received the same amount of pressure, i.e. that it is completely vertical, it fires a large needle into the middle of the sternum where it meets the centre of the bone, an excellent way of then introducing drugs and fluids into the patient. Seconds later, we had access, and with a quick eye contact from Inky, a meet with The Pope was scheduled for later that day.

A brief pause in chest compressions facilitated a carotid pulse check. Kieran's concentration intensified and he leaned a little closer to Delroy. A quick glance at the cardiac monitor confirmed his suspicions that we'd got a pulse back and a cardiac output. He quietly voiced his findings to the rest of us. More drugs and fluids continued and I sorted getting Delroy out of the flat and into the waiting ambulance that had also attended. The guys travelled with Delroy to hospital. His cardiac rhythm had stabilised but he continued to need ventilating. The hospital was alerted and a convoy of emergency vehicles proceeded to the nearest hospital being given the cursory police motorcycle escort arranged some short time previously. Having been handed over to the waiting hospital staff, we all got our kit together, cleaned up and readied for a debrief in the car with a maxpax coffee.

Debriefing is a vital part of pretty much any job big or small, and whether it's a cosy affair between a crew in an ambulance or car after the job or a more formal affair between all the services taking place in a conference room, they form a vital part of the learning process. Who did what, when and what went well or could be improved? It's a reflective process that allows us to examine our practice and how we can keep what went well and change what didn't, as in the heat of the moment we do what we think is the right thing but in hind sight it may not have been. Aside of a few elements in Delroy's case we jointly decided that the case went reasonably well but that the likelihood was that Delroy would either not survive or would be severely brain damaged due to the length of time his brain would have been deprived of oxygen. This sat well with us because it was an element to which we'd had no control. For us, the case was filed with all the other cases to be a thing of the past by the end of the shift. Rarely did I ever get the opportunity to follow up on cases such as this. Daniel Beechdale had been one, and this was another.

Nearly a year later, I attended a rehabilitation unit in Birmingham. It was a new build place for predominantly stroke victims who attended for their journey back to health. Here they could get specialised physiotherapy, speech therapy and help with learning how to walk, dress, wash and generally survive back in the world. I had been tasked to pick up a patient and take him to a home residential address for weekend 'leave', as was so often the case with patients from this unit gaining some time to reacquaint themselves with returning to home life, but needing ambulance assistance to facilitate the journey. The address I was to take the patient to didn't ring a bell and I hadn't been there before. Even the name didn't initially spike my attention when I read it on the sheet. That was until I saw the patient; Delroy.

He looked so different. Half the weight, different hair style and an absence of bling, and despite only having been a year since his cardiac arrest, he looked 10 years older. He struggled with standing unaided and certainly couldn't walk instead relying on a wheelchair. His face was contorted and semi paralysed and his one hand was bent towards his body and tucked into his torso, clearly having no ability to use it. The cursory chat and introduction to him revealed a speech which was difficult to understand, and left a constant dribble down his chin and wetted his tee shirt. It wasn't until this journey that I became aware of Delroy's story, and at the time I'd attended his hanging, it was just another story-less hanging. But keen to know his details I engaged him in conversation and he was only too happy to tell me the tale. I didn't feel it appropriate to let him know I'd been at his cardiac arrest; do you become the hero for bringing him back into this world with severe disability, or the arsehole that has done so? I was left with the distinct impression that he had never intended to commit suicide and that it was just a plan that went wrong. His disability wasn't just confined to his paralysis either. He now suffered fits, emotional and concentration issues and would clearly need supervision for the rest of his life. Of course, he didn't win the heart of Sam back either, and hadn't seen her since the incident. Another part of his life to alter forever.

CHAPTER 32.
JUMPING ON THE BANDWAGON

By 2008 the mid life crisis was well under way and had worked itself into my private life. Now it was time for it to spread its wings into the workplace. I'd been tutoring in ambulance training school since 2000 and despite loving the job was beginning to find it a little tedious. Teaching for the duration of an ambulance technician or paramedic course provided enough variety on a day-to-day basis to be enjoyable and keep me motivated. But one-day update programmes consisting of the same daily content over and over again for weeks on end became draining. We all had to do our bit, and none of us relished our turn. Gaining the opportunity to branch out to educate within the university environment gave a different perspective and was good for my resumé. This was the inauguration and conceptive time of the move from in house training to university based education, and brought with it a whole plethora of change.

Teaching delivery would from this time forward, be performed using a holistic approach of not only paramedic science, but nursing skills and under pinning knowledge too, so now nurses could build upon the students academic base. The practical on-road element would now be more structured and mentor based. This was one area that most of the tutors looked forward to. It was an opportunity to get out of the classroom for a few days, get back on the road, and interact with the patient. A sort of 'return to grass roots' style of working, and consisted of either crewing up with a student or riding shotgun with a crew to be able to offer guidance and support to paramedic fledgelings. But it wasn't without its pitfalls. Sometimes it was like pushing shit uphill with some of the more challenging guys, who struggled with the practical elements and a breeze with the easy ones who took to it like a duck to water.

One such student was Stefan Skinner, an intelligent lad who'd developed an impatience to gain the paramedic qualification and was deeply pissed off that if he'd have been on the last course, he would not have had to jump through the hoops he now had to for the next year, and could have qualified under the old scheme in a matter of a few months. So his course was the first of the new ones. Initially, Stefan hadn't impressed me because of his attitude and approach to the course, and found himself in hot water on more than one occasion for not toeing the line in defiance. His body language was often the child stood in the corner, arms folded, stamping feet and wingeing about anything and everything. He just didn't seem to get the fact that he couldn't change the time scale, or the elements of the course that he found insultingly easy. In his defence, he was experienced in both pre hospital care and life, and his reasoning was always sound, but there was still no other way forward. It was lighting the blue touch paper and standing well back when, for example, he sat through a lecture on an element of pre hospital care, such as trauma assessment, by a nurse who'd never set foot outside of the hospital, and whose only clinical experience had been gained from a urology ward! Did he give the lecturer a hard time or what? To the point I felt sorry for the guy, as Stefan used academia and superior knowledge for the purpose of slaughter. I could completely understand his issue. But none of us could change things, and he would just have to accept it.

As the months passed however, Stefan mellowed and accepted that he had to serve his time. He still expressed his annoyance but settled and became easier and less irritating to teach and mentor. As I got to know him better, I started to warm to him, and found him sharing his home life details with me. He'd served in the British army, which endears a particular sense of humour I like, and find funny, but I realised that a soldiers approach being one of 'change something if it isn't right' was the problem. His frustration was borne out of this inability to change something that he considered wasn't right. But his acceptance of things was then the product of 'adapt and overcome'.

As his year progressed, the theory input reduced, and was replaced with on-road practical mentoring, consisting of one-on-one working with a tutor to gain an agreed amount of hours of supervised operational placement. Stef was an easy student to mentor. Now he had the paramedic skills and was able to use them under my supervision, he flourished, and was good at his job, to the point where when he was in the back with the patient, he'd shout through to me driving to tell me he was about to perform a particular procedure, or administer a drug, rather than ask me. He had become autonomous; a sure sign he was ready for independent practice.

February 2009 saw Stef on his final few mentor shifts and I was covering them. It wasn't like working with a student, but more like with an old colleague with loads of years under his belt. I looked forward to working with him because of his manner and competence now being a pleasure to work with. I left the house early and drove over to his base station in Shrewsbury meeting up with him for a day shift of 0700 to 1900 hrs. It was an old building that had been used as an ambulance station since the year dot, reminding me of Henrietta Street in central Birmingham. It was a bit like that old ragged pullover that really needed throwing out but was just too comfortable to do so.

The day started out very much as an ordinary shift. A collapse, doctor's urgent admission into Hospital, a maternity case, a simple trauma and an elderly male unwell, taking us up to mid afternoon. We'd taken the old chap into the emergency department and had a brew while Stef completed the paperwork. I couldn't help but notice that while we'd been in the department, there had been an awful lot of noise and commotion in the resuscitation room, with people coming and going, but always the curtains being drawn upon anyone's entry or exit. Being one of only two ambulances covering the area, I knew we hadn't brought anything in, so both back in the ambulance, I asked Stef if he knew anything about the patient.

"So what's the score with the commotion in resus then Stef?" His preoccupation with finalising the paperwork from the last job, meant a slight delay in his reply. His pen back in the sleeve pocket and, starring forward, he replied.

"Oh yeah, I heard all that panic too. I asked Jane what the score was and apparently it's a 10 year old cardiac arrest that they got back."

"10 year old?" I quizzed, looking at him. "Bloody hell. I'm guessing a drowning or a pre existing." Stef continued.

"Not difficult to guess is it on someone that young. Known epileptic, fitted in the garden and fell into the fish pond unnoticed. By the time his mother found him, he'd been down a while Jane reckons. She told us to expect to transfer him later if he survives that long." The conversation ended with a comment from me.

"Well that'll be a nice little job to finish us off then." Brilliant. With an hours drive back home and now likely to finish on time, I'd be home in front of the fire for quarter past eight. But as the saying goes. If something's guaranteed, it rarely comes off.

Stef pressed the 'clear at hospital' button on our MDT (mobile data terminal) in the ambulance, and we sat in silence for a few moments waiting for the next job which was likely our nice little transfer to the bigger general hospital up the road, and with collecting and delivering the patient, even though it was local, it would still take about an hour and a half, taking us, I estimated, to about 1830, then a return to station to hand over to the night crew who would jump early for us if a job came in. Sorted. Well not quite. The MDT bleeped and Stef scrolled a message asking us to contact control by phone. Experience should have told me, not to bank on finishing on time. Whenever control ask to speak on the phone, they have something time consuming going on. Stef jumped out of the truck.

"Back in a sec...." The door slammed and he walked back into the casualty dept to make the call, returning about five minutes later. He'd got a look on his face that I couldn't read. "D'ya fancy some overtime?" He asked. Rarely did I ever turn down overtime, but occasionally if a bottle of Merlot had my name on it, a refusal got serious consideration.

"Well, I'd rather not, but what's up?" He stood in the open doorway of the ambulance, poised as if ready to spring into action.

"I don't think you'll turn this one down. The kid in resus needs urgent transfer, and the nearest ITU bed is Liverpool, and there's no one else to do it if we don't. Clearly that's going to take us over finishing time, so they're asking if we'll do it." The merlot would have to wait. Some things are more important. Before I could tell him all was good, he came back

"And there's more. He keeps re arresting. 10 times so far. The doc is hoping to stabilise him, and as soon as he is, doc wants to go, and wants a real flyer to Liverpool without the delay of calling for us to come back. He wants us to stand by here until the moment he's ready, then we go."

"And are control ok with that?" I asked.

"Yeah, it's cool. They're gonna try and get the night shift to come in early. Anyway, everyone knows that if we don't do it this way, the poor bugger won't survive. Not with the lack of paediatric skill they have here. He has to go out. It's just a shit that the nearest fuckin' bed is so far away. Bloody state of the NHS."

My look told Stef I was up for it and he disappeared back into the department to let control know. I got the stretcher off and took it into the resus room, where there was still a flurry of excitement. Standing at the head of the patient, the doctor was on the phone clearly discussing the patient with the receiving doctor for Liverpool, some 120 miles away. The patient had tubes, cannulas and wires into seemingly every orifice and vein in his little body. His eyes were taped shut and his breathing was automated via a ventilator and an intubation tube was sticking out of his mouth. His chest rose sharply every few seconds, and the cardiac monitor bleeped away next to him with an erratic rhythm taking place. 3 or 4 nurses approached him, did something, then went away, sometimes out of the room returning seconds later with some other piece of kit or drug, drawn up ready in a syringe. Another nurse stood in the corner writing and recording everything. They all seemed to work as a well oiled team.

The doctor finished his phone call, adjusted the ventilator then turned to me.

"Hi guys. Thanks for coming so promptly. I'm Dr Stevens. This young man needs to go to The Children's Hospital in Liverpool as it's the nearest bed we can find. He's pretty poorly at the moment and keeps arresting. We've been going for about 30 minutes so far since the last, and fingers crossed he's beginning to improve......" His words tailed off as one of the monitors alarms started bleeping, and the team heightened their attention towards the patient again. Clearly in the way for now, I decided to back away. The doc would know where to find us when the time was right.

In contrast to popular public belief, fed by adventurous media-ship, the majority of emergency calls never necessitated insane speeds to get to the patient. However, we never know how serious a case is until we can front up to the scene. And only then do we conclude that 80% of all calls didn't need an emergency response. As a consequence, very few cases need a speedy journey into hospital. But some do, and this was one of them. Before the days of satellite navigation, to assist the smooth passage through to hospital, we used to have the facility of The Police to provide an escort, which was great if we were off area and didn't know where we were going. The principle was for a police vehicle, car or motorcycle, to travel in front of the ambulance, with lights and sirens activated, to create a pathway through the traffic, and thus allowing a faster passage to the destination. If done properly, it allowed the ambulance the facility of a constant speed; not having to accelerate or brake, even if the speed was only 20 to 30 miles an hour, meant an improved outcome to someone who had a spinal injury for example, and a much easier working environment for those in the back of the moving ambulance, which can be a pretty busy workplace under these conditions.

I rang the control room, in the vein hope of arranging the escort.

"Hi Fran, it's Dave. Look, with ref to this kiddy transfer, we've got a bit of an issue....." My words tailed off as she pre-empted my query.

"I know what you're gonna say," she started. "You don't know how to get to Liverpool Children's do you? I continued.

"Well, man of many talents I may be, but a geographical guru I am not. So, any chance you can ring the cops and see if they can organise an escort for us?" Her short hesitation in reply said it all. I knew we'd have difficulty in sorting something out. Fran went on.

"Dave, the police are getting funny lately about doing escorts, so it's doubtful but I'll try."

"Cheers Fran, you're a star. But with the state of this poor lad, if I don't know the route, it's going to be bloody detrimental."

Stef and I sat in the front of the ambulance in silence. To start, things were fine. As the driver for this case, I was trying to sort my route from some old map books I'd managed to get hold of. This was before the era of Google maps and navigation. But as the minutes, then hours dragged on, boredom set in. We had to be ready to go within one minutes notice, so only trips to the loo were permitted. No canteen breaks, and no wandering about.

The silence was broken by the familiar ring of my mobile phone. It was Fran, and her tone didn't sound hopeful.

"Hey Dave, look.....the police said they don't have the resourcing to help. But a really helpful bloke there made some calls and got back to me. Apparently the Mersey Tunnel Police will pick you up from the far side of the tunnel and will take you to the hospital as a pilot only. So you've only got to find your way to the Mersey Tunnel which should make life a little easier."

"Ah great", I replied. "Well that's better than nothing. Thanks Fran".

A 'pilot' escort was merely a police or other vehicle who remained in front of the ambulance, but who knew the route. So following them was like having a personal guide. That in itself was good. But often the pilot was an unmarked vehicle with no emergency lights or sirens, and often nobody trained to drive under emergency conditions either. This meant that we'd hot drive up as far as the pilot, then we'd have to switch everything off to pootle behind him for the remainder of the journey. The advantage of the escort would be counteracted by having to drive that last part at normal legal speeds. A pain in the arse if this poor boy was continuing to arrest on a regular basis. And an arrest in the back of an ambulance meant no extra nurses to help, no fancy drugs aside of those brought along, and no senior doctor backup apart from the one that was coming with us. Instead, this mobile casualty room would provide few resources, poor light, and limited ability to get the child back from The Reaper. So any delays would not be good. The call to Fran ended and following updating Stef, the silence resumed.

I'd started to feel irritated. I needed sustenance and all that was on offer was machine coffee; its bitter, gritty taste revolted me but I decided it was better than nothing....just. Besides, I'd started to get boredom sleepy, and that wasn't a good idea. It was nearing 7pm and I was hoping that we'd get the call sooner rather than later. Stef's folded arms supported his drooping chin. Head pitched forward, his soft rhythmical snoring repeatedly broke the silence. Then came a tap on the window of the ambulance, and Stef shot up in surprise, simultaneously wiping his mouth with the back of his hand and stretching in one movement. He wound down the window, and an excitable young nurse spoke up.

"We're on guys. The boy has been stable now for over an hour". She left not waiting for a reply and Stef jumped out to follow. I called up on the radio to let them know, then followed.

Having left the stretcher in the emergency department, the team had already loaded the patient onto it. The usual process with unstable transfers is to load the patient then wait before leaving in the ambulance just to see if the stability remains, as just moving a patient is often destabilising. I was expecting to move there and then. But the furore of activity brought it home that that point still hadn't quite arrived. Here was this patient, emanating tubes and wires, drip pumps aplenty injecting drugs and fluid into several veins. An automatic respirator clipped onto the side of the stretcher rhythmically filled his chest with air, creating that classic and familiar sound of a ventilated child. There wasn't a spare inch of room on the stretcher that didn't have something on it. And weeping at the head end was a distraught mother. Yesterday, she was scolding him for being late home. Yesterday she hugged him good night. Yesterday, he finished his paper round early so he could go out with his mates. And now all that was a distant memory as she watched and felt the life slipping out of him. The next few hours would become her worst nightmare. And the next hour or so would become a challenge for Stef and myself too.

I'd studied the doctor, who in turn had all his focus on the monitors, for several minutes. He was clearly anxious and didn't at all seem relaxed. He'd developed a nervous finger movement on the side of his face and bit his lip with anxiety, as he stood motionless watching. Just watching. After a while he turned to me.

"Right chaps, there's no time like the present. Here's the plan....." He'd captivated both our attention. "We'll do this in stages. First, we'll move him to the ambulance, we load him, then we monitor and we wait. I reckon about 20 minutes. Then, if he remains stable, we go. And if he arrests again, we'll divert to the nearest A and E. Happy?" Stef grabbed the far end of the stretcher and I replied

"Right o doc. Routes' sorted, and we're all good to go." The team readied and rallied around the young boy, and I tried to imagine the muddle going through the docs head. While he was in the comfort of the ED, he'd got everything; light, staff, back up, communication, drugs, power and confidence. Once on the road however, he'd have few of this if the shit hit the fan. Welcome to my world.

The monitor's beeping continued with an encouraging regularity and the alarms didn't go off. But we all knew this boy had so far to go, as the stretcher was gently wheeled out of the room towards the waiting ambulance. It felt like we'd got a priceless artefact in our care. Some multi million pound fragile piece of art work. And I guess to his mum, we did.

The doors to the back of the ambulance opened and in we all went for the next stage of the waiting and monitoring game. Doctor Stevens and one of the nurses were travelling with us, along with a plethora of gear; boxes of equipment and bags of drugs, to the point where there wasn't any more room for anything or anybody else. Stef and I stayed out and before closing the doors reminded the team to shout up if they needed anything. But our words fell on deaf ears. Their focus was elsewhere.

It's at times like this that no matter how experienced or professional one is, humanism comes in to play. If I'd have been a smoker, pacing up and down the side of the ambulance drawing deeply upon the cigarette wouldn't have looked out of place, and I really expected things to go wrong, and we'd all be rushing back inside the ED. But, unexpectedly, the back door opened and a head popped out wearing a mildly confident look. My imaginary smoke now dropped onto the pile already on the floor, followed by my foot stamping and twisting it out. I looked up.

"Let's go chaps. He's stable. For the moment at least".

I fired up the engine and with a final confirmatory head nod from the doc in my interior mirror, we headed off with blue lights intermittently illuminating the now dark trees lining the exit from the hospital. Stef sat in the front. With the speed and delicacy needed for this trip, a second pair of eyes on the road was very welcome, as was a navigator. Making a wrong turn when out for a Sunday picnic doesn't usually carry a life threat. This journey however was entirely different. Settling in, I tried to concentrate solely on the driving, letting Stef keep a check on how things were going in the back. Even so, I couldn't help but be aware of the situation. Whilst the two of them remained seated, things were good. Standing up and leaning over the patient from time to time, however, put my blood pressure up slightly, and invariably Stef's pulse rate, as I saw his hand slide down towards the release button on his seat belt in preparation of jumping in the back to assist, only to cease his plan as the doc sat down again, having pressed another button or adjusted one of the many syringe drivers.

Our journey was to take us up the A49, then further north onto the A41 and then up the M53 to the Mersey Tunnel to pick up our pilot. Ambulance control had already confirmed there to be no known road works or delays on this route, and the further we got into it, the more I relaxed, trying to keep a balance between progression and a smooth drive. Straight sections allowed more speed, overtaking slower vehicles, and plotting gaps to gently weave around the cars. Blue flashing lights at night, and in the darkness help to be seen, and drivers showed welcome courtesy to us, allowing the guys in the rear to get on with their constant attention to detail without being thrown around. Roundabouts were negotiated slowly and with the straightest pathway, having used forward vision and anticipation of other road users, to then accelerate with silkiness. Ever onwards into the darkness of the A roads, getting nearer and nearer to our destination.

Up onto the motorway saw me mouth some thanks to be saying goodbye to the traffic islands and overtakes that had adorned the main roads in Shropshire, as now I could increase the speed a little. Stef occasionally spoke up to ask if all was good in the back, and Doc Stevens confirmed things to be fine at each occasion, as we continued to breathe some slight sighs of relief. Often in similar circumstances, idle chat takes over; questions of what the weekend hails, did you get your car fixed or statements of how hungry one was just seemed so inappropriate, and I was glad Stef remained quiet. My concentration was just too intense. And then, as now, I have an inability to multi-task. So aside of the occasional question aimed backwards, Stef's only other words were confirmatory remarks of the road conditions; clear to the left, clear to the right, safe to proceed through this or that junction and so on. As the pressure was on, I welcomed every word.

Fran in Comms had asked me earlier to give them a call when we were about five miles out from the tunnel so the pilot could make ready. Choosing a point, where, at about 90mph, there was little traffic in front of us, I piped up and broke the silence.

"Stef, give control a call will ya, and let 'em know we're about five miles out from the tunnel entrance?" He instinctively obeyed without acknowledgment.

"Metro 164 over." He spoke into the mic. After being advised to continue, he carried on. "164, we're approaching five miles out from the tunnel entrance. Can you inform the pilot that we'll be with him in about 10 minutes over".

"Yes roger that 164," came the reply. "Will do. Metro out".

Within minutes, as we approached the on ramp of a junction, I became aware of a police traffic car parked on the hard shoulder, half way down the ramp. As we sped past it, my inside door mirror picked up the noticeable flashing of its blue lights previously not on. I hadn't connected us with it, and just assumed by coincidence, the guys had got a job just as we came past. We were, after all still a way out from our pilot, who was probably, I'd imagined, a plain transit van, as the tunnel police often use. Watching him in my mirror, he picked up speed quickly, moving in first behind us as he crossed lanes, then overtaking us before dropping in front some 100 metres ahead. I soon realised, that he was escorting us into the tunnel as the signs for it rapidly approached before skimming overhead. Being now 9pm, the traffic was still light, but what a difference the escort did make to what was in front of us. Car after car in lane three moved across for the traffic car, allowing us safe and speedy passage through.

We entered the tunnel and the over head lights lit everything up, making vision so much better. Further and further we drove, but looking forward, I struggled to see our pilot waiting. Perhaps he wasn't going to be there? If the motorway police tailed off at the end of the tunnel leaving us, we were in the shit, and would have to rely on good old fashioned maps. My anxiety rose, as I knew ours to be out of date. Heading towards the middle of a big city, travelling at speed, without a clue where we were, wasn't the place to be right now. One wrong lane, or missed sign would mean potentially heading up some motorway, completely in the wrong direction looking for an exit which would take us even further away. Then the issue of getting onto Control, telling them where we were, waiting for replies and phone calls to make to get help, if it was even available. My mind went into freak mode. Fortunately I managed the swan syndrome; that ability to visual remain calm and collected above the water, while all along your legs are working to a blur to keep the forward propulsion. I broke the silence with a hushed voice so the guys in the back wouldn't hear.

"I sure hope to fuck, these coppers don't leave us if the bloody pilot isn't there." In my peripheral vision I could see Stef's face give a wry smile before he replied.

"We're on the same wave length there brother......" His words tailing off as the darker end of the tunnel in front signified its end. If only we could have spoken directly to the guys in the motorway patrol car in front. But we needn't have worried. As if from nowhere a second set of blue lights appeared from another car in front that had been stationary on the side of the road in a lay-by near the exit. Before we had chance to approach, it too accelerated with speed so there were now two in front of us. My pulse rate subsided slightly with some relief, as we came out of the lit tunnel and into the yellow fluorescence of the street lighting on the main road that was to take us into the city. As the road rose up the incline I slowed a little to negotiate the upcoming brow. The first car in front disappeared over it, followed by the second and then us, with them reappearing as soon as the road had flattened out.

As I counted them back in again, I had to look twice, as there were now three sets of blue lights. Then four, and five. It seemed like everyone wanted to come out and play, and as we rounded the next corner, the first few cars had positioned themselves to block anyone access from some side roads onto the main highway, effectively allowing us to not have to slow for these junctions. This was turning out to be somewhat adrenaline fuelled, but little did we know it was to get better. Up ahead from us, was what looked like a road block. A sea of flashing blue strobes blending into one. As we neared them, I could make out several police motorcycles, so many in number, I couldn't count, and parked on both sides of the road on our side of the duel carriageway.

Before we could reach them, they'd all shot off into the distance, already, individually starting to block every road, traffic island, petrol station and driveway that threatened us with a vehicle pulling out and slowing our progression. Each bike or car we passed, would be seen to accelerate up behind us, then overtake on either side to join the queue in front for their next task, engines screaming as they did. Bikes would come past us on a bend at such speed and angle of lean it was reminiscent of my motorcycle track days. Sirens would get louder very quickly, then lower their tone as they blitzed past us. The police cars by now were having difficulty in keeping up, aside of the one that had originally picked us up on the motorway, and whose job now was to remain directly in front of us keeping our speed at a constant and remain in contact with all the others in the escort, slowing or increasing speed slightly depending on the information relayed back to him from the guys at the front. Cars had the top speed alright, but not the sheer unadulterated acceleration or the nimbleness of the motorcycles.

Junction after junction, roundabout after roundabout were negotiated with safety and ease. And to help out further, some hazards even had foot police standing blocking access to our pathway. I'd been involved with police escorts on many previous occasions, but I'd never seen such an organised and well manned operation, that was probably arranged in a very short time.

My concentration had been such as to give me the luxury of forgetting what was happening in the rear, aside of getting them to our destination. Several expletives had also emanated from Stef's mouth as we progressed further. Relatively hushed words of "fuck me," and "Jesus, that was bloody close!", were almost in synchronisation as we marvelled at the skill afforded to us. Lefts and rights then started getting more often and the roads became narrower, and I knew we weren't far away from our target. Then the signs telling us we were only a mile away were relayed into the rear so the guys could start to breathe easier.

I slowed the vehicle down to a crawl as we pulled into the hospital entrance and brought us to a stop under the canopy of the doors. Handbrake on, I took a second to exhale. In that second, the bikes, cars, blue lights, sirens, speed and adrenaline disappeared as quickly as they had come. In a puff of someone's magic lantern they were gone. And we were here. At the hospital, having been teleported safely and smoothly. Our patient had remained stable, and with a noisy sigh I turned off the engine and prepared to move our boy to his intensive care.

This was another of the many cases that I never chased up to know the outcome of this poor boy. I often like to be positive and think, that now, some 16 years on, he's a healthy 26 year old, doing what 26 year olds do; drinking, womanising and working. What made it possible? The vigilance and skill of Doctor Stevens and his team of nurses, and the organisation and sheer ability of the Merseyside Police. Looking back, I'm certain that this had been a blast for them. In Birmingham in years gone by, we never had to ask the bike cops twice to give us an escort. They loved it. But the escorting process was seen by the health and safety bods as being too risky and unnecessary, and like with so many good things, was lost to 'progress'.

This was to have been my last shift working for an NHS Ambulance Service, and although I did several more teaching days, no more would I take the pulse or check the blood pressure of a patient on English soil as a full time employed paramedic. What a job to finish on though! From my first ever case as a front line clinician dealing with the four dead in the head on collision in Hockley, Birmingham, some 22 years before, to this exciting police escort, and everything in between. What a rollercoaster.

CHAPTER 33. AND FINALLY.....

As of 2025, the average career term of a paramedic is a little over five years. So the masses of young people qualifying from universities and looking to start their lives as prehospital carers barely covers the vacancies created.

Perhaps those paramedics that leave around the five year mark are the lucky ones. Maybe they see something that I never did. If they go on to work in another profession which doesn't involve shift work, endangerment, threats, stress, lack of sleep, poor eating habits and cortisol coming out of their ears on a frequent basis, then maybe they won't experience the not-so-nice side of the job. I, like so many of my colleagues who've served for many years, have gone through more than one divorce, have had more than my fair share of mental health issues, and have used alcohol as an escape for many years. But on the other side of the coin, I wouldn't have had it any other way. My career has shaped me to the people pleaser I am, and it's humbling to have been able to provide that prehospital care to the thousands of individuals who have either breathed their last breath in my arms or gone on to stick the V's up to the reaper.

Two books I've recently read, *Unnatural Causes* by Dr Richard Shepherd, and *Undoctored* by Adam Kay, himself an ex doctor by choice, both exert just what the provision of health care at the sharp end can do to the care givers.

My eldest daughter, Emily, is a paramedic in New Zealand, working as an educator and clinical support officer. She too is exposed to what I am, and I worry about her mental health. Fortunately, modern ambulance services are far more aware of MH issues and provide for counselling and talking things through at a professional level. It seems incomprehensible that 30 years ago following attending the poor bloke cut in half under the train, and being shot at through the windscreen of the ambulance and nearly being beheaded by machete, that we just carried on regardless, without a thought for how that may have affected us in the long run.

Ever since I can remember, in working for an ambulance service, staffing has always been a problem. There has just never been enough people to man the vehicles. I think this is a combination of several factors. The media has for decades now, portrayed the life of a paramedic as a very dramatic one; road accident, after stabbing, after shooting, after cardiac arrest. The truth however is somewhat more mundane, with 'bread and butter' cases of low acuity scenarios forming 90% of our working days. This, coupled with a massive increase in verbal and physical assaults on ambulance staff has seen a great deal of staff members become disillusioned and as a consequence, change careers and move away.

The public perception of the service that pre-hospital care offers has also dramatically changed. Gone are the days in the 1980's and before, that fractured ankles, bumped heads and bleeding injuries would be put in the family car and self transported to hospital. Now we see ambulances attending the mildly unwell, the individuals who live opposite the hospital entrances, and the downright bizarre cases of the stubbed toes and the broken fingernails. There can't be a paramedic anywhere in the world with a bit of service under their belts who hasn't been called to the elderly in need of the channel changing on the television. There is just such a greater expectation of the ambulance services, and all too often we encompass an attitude of entitlement. The public we see often just don't seem to be able to sort out their minor slips, trips and dribbly dicks.

Of course, there is also an increasing population, and who are living to a greater age, all putting strain on medical services as a whole. Where the hospital emergency department can't release a cubicle because there isn't a bed upstairs available for the patient, so the ambulance crew can't unload the next patient into that cubicle, meaning the unfortunately injured remains on the ambulance stretcher, and which produces one less ambulance to attend the next emergency call about to come in. It's a vicious circle.

This has meant that the amount of overtime worked by paramedics to cover the basic rostering has always been, and always will be, immense. The donkey will work harder if there is reward, until such time as exhaustion causes him to fall over. Paramedics the world over, who work in busy areas, namely the cities, work 12 hour shifts, often without breaks, and more often end their shifts with late cases. With the commute to and from work, this means around only nine to 10 hours between shifts in a run of four days. That's nine hours to eat, sleep and spend time with the family. No wonder so many seek to exchange this type of work for something less exhausting.

In 2007, Australian ambulance services, unable to fill their vacancy needs from within the country, out sourced and advertised in the UK for paramedics. Offering better money, enhanced working conditions, awesome weather and an overall improvement in lifestyle, they advertised in medical publications and in person at international pre-hospital care conferences.

I turned up at a friend's place sometime in mid 2007 to be met with an enormous map of Australia on the wall. I'd known

Karl for many years and worked alongside him as a paramedic. We shared a love of Landrovers and all things off roading. He informed me that he had applied to work for The Queensland Ambulance Service and had been accepted, and suggested I should look into it too. Just like all those years ago, when Mary made the preposterous suggestion to apply to work in the ambulance service, now too, Karl was suggesting an equally stupid move which I initially gave little to no thought about. However, yet again, from many an acorn grows an oak tree, and before long I found myself applying, passing the tests and interviews, and on April 1st 2009, boarding a British Airways flight to Brisbane. And so the next chapter of my life had begun.

Just like some 22 years before, what I was about to let myself in for I had no idea. No idea of the characters I would meet, or the circumstances I would find myself in. Giant spiders, snake bites, vast distances and people as hard as coffin nails would be crossing my path expecting me to deal with them and sort out their problems. 16 years later however, these people and events have given me more experiences to share with you.

EPILOGUE

Thank you for taking the time to read my book and allow me to share my tales. I hope that you've gained at least a few laughs, and perhaps shed the odd tear, as I have done. One of my intentions was to give an insight into at least a little of my world as a paramedic over the years, and how things have changed. This book catalogues nearly 40 years of experiences, and has been 12 years in the making, setting out with the intention of providing myself some form of self-counselling, as I find that writing not only soothes the soul, but allows one to express, relive, examine, construct, criticise and reveal in a way that speaking cannot. Words can be taken back, altered and pondered on before being presented to the reader only when the writer is ready, and that suits me.

Having worked alone for most of my 38 years as an ambo, I have had less chance for that vital counselling that takes place between ambulance crews following harrowing cases. In 2014 I went through some mental turmoil and PTSD that spurned me to start my literary musings in an attempt for this self help. I started writing this book well after I'd emigrated, and now, across the dusty roads and remote corners of the Aussie outback, I've met a whole new cast of characters; wild, wonderful, tragic and hilarious, and their stories deserve to be told, listened to and read.

So, if you've enjoyed '*A Paramedic's Daze*', look out for the next exciting Aussie phase, '***Ambo Dave***'.

To be continued.....

www.ingramcontent.com/pod-product-compliance
Lightning Source LLC
Chambersburg PA
CBHW071648090426
42738CB00009B/1452